Workbook
prepared by

Jean Giddens, RN, MS, CS
Assistant Professor of Nursing
Nursing and Radiological Sciences
Mesa State College
Grand Junction, Colorado

Textbook

Sharon Mantik Lewis, RN, PhD, FAAN
Professor, College of Nursing
Research Associate Professor, Department of Pathology
University of New Mexico
Albuquerque, New Mexico

Margaret McLean Heitkemper, RN, PhD, FAAN
Professor, Biobehavioral Nursing and Health Systems
School of Nursing
University of Washington
Seattle, Washington

Shannon Ruff Dirksen, RN, PhD
Associate Professor, College of Nursing
Arizona State University
Tempe, Arizona

Contents

Part VIII—Problems Related to Movement and Coordination

Getting Started

GETTING SET UP

■ MINIMUM SYSTEM REQUIREMENTS

Virtual Clinical Excursions is a hybrid CD, so it runs on both Macintosh and Windows platforms. To use *Virtual Clinical Excursions*, you will need one of the following systems:

- **Windows™**

  Windows 2000, 95, 98, NT 4.0
  IBM compatible computer
  Pentium II processor (or equivalent)
  300 MHz
  96 MB
  800 × 600 screen size
  256 color monitor
  100 MB hard drive space
  12× CD-ROM drive
  Soundblaster 16 soundcard compatibility
  Stereo speakers or headphones

- **Macintosh®**

  MAC OS 9.04
  Apple Power PC G3
  300 MHz
  96 MB
  800 × 600 screen size
  256 color monitor
  100 MB hard drive space
  12× CD-ROM drive
  Stereo speakers or headphones

Ideally, the system you use should have at least 200 MB of free disk space on your hard drive. There are commercially available desktop utility programs that can help clean up your hard drive. No other applications besides the operating system should be running at the time *Virtual Clinical Excursions* is running.

1

■ INSTALLING *VIRTUAL CLINICAL EXCURSIONS*

Virtual Clinical Excursions is designed to run from a set of files on your hard drive and a CD in your CD-ROM. Minimal installation is required.

- **Windows™**

  1. Start Microsoft Windows and insert *Virtual Clinical Excursions* **Disk 1 (Installation)** in the CD-ROM drive.
  2. Click the **Start** icon on the taskbar and select the **Run** option.
  3. Type d:\setup.exe (where "d:\" is your CD-ROM drive) and press OK.
  4. Follow the on-screen instructions for installation.
  5. Remove *Virtual Clinical Excursions* **Disk 1 (Installation)** from your CD-ROM drive.
  6. Restart your computer.

- **Macintosh®**

  1. Insert *Virtual Clinical Excursions* **Disk 1 (Installation)** in the CD-ROM drive. The disk icon will appear on your desktop.
  2. Double-click on the disk icon.
  3. Double-click on the icon **Install Virtual Clinical Excursions**.
  4. Follow the on-screen instructions for installation.
  5. Remove *Virtual Clinical Excursions* **Disk 1 (Installation)** from your CD-ROM drive
  6. Restart your computer.

■ HOW TO RESET YOUR MONITOR TO 256 COLORS

This software will only run if the monitor is set at 256 colors. To reset your monitor:

- **Windows™**

  1. Choose **Settings** from the **Start** menu.
  2. Choose **Control Panel**.
  3. Double-click on the **Display** icon.
  4. Click on the **Settings** tab.
  5. In the **Colors** drop-down menu, click on the arrow to show more settings.
  6. Click on **256 Colors**.
  7. Click on **Apply**.
  8. Click on **OK**.
  9. If the system asks whether you wish to restart your computer to accept these settings, click on **Yes**.

- **Macintosh®**

  1. Choose the **Monitors** control panel.
  2. Change the color display to **256**.

■ **HOW TO USE DISK 2 (PATIENTS' DISK)**

- **Windows™**

  When you want to work with the five patients in the virtual hospital, follow these steps:

  1. Insert *Virtual Clinical Excursions* **Disk 2 (Patients' Disk)** into your CD-ROM drive.
  2. Double-click on the icon **Shortcut to Virtual Clinical Excursions**, which can be found on your desktop. This will load and run the program.

- **Macintosh®**

  When you want to work with the five patients in the virtual hospital, follow these steps:

  1. Insert *Virtual Clinical Excursions* **Disk 2 (Patients' Disk)** into your CD-ROM drive.
  2. Double-click on the icon **Shortcut to Virtual Clinical Excursions**, which can be found on your desktop. This will load and run the program.

■ **QUALITY OF VISUALS, SPEED, AND COMMON PROBLEMS**

Virtual Clinical Excursions uses the Apple QuickTime media layer system. This includes Quick-Time Video and QuickTime VR Video, which allow for high-quality graphics and digital video. The graphics seen in the *Virtual Clinical Excursions* courseware should be of high quality with good color. If the movies and graphics appear blocky or otherwise low-quality, check to see whether your video card is set to "thousands of colors."

Note: Virtual Clinical Excursions is not designed to function at a 256-color depth. (You may need to go to the Control Panel and change the Display settings.) If you don't see any digital video options, please check that QuickTime is installed correctly.

The system should respond quickly and smoothly. In particular, you should not see any jerky motions or unannounced long delays as you move through the virtual hospital settings, interact with patients, or access information resources. If you notice slow, jerky, or delayed software responses, it may mean that your particular system requires additional RAM, your processor does not meet the basic requirements, or your hard drive is full or too fragmented. If the videos appear banded or subject to "breakup," you may need to find an updated video driver for the computer's video card. Please consult the manufacturer of the video card or computer for additional video drivers for your machine.

■ **TECHNICAL SUPPORT**

Technical support for this product is available at no charge by calling the Technical Support Hotline between 9 a.m. and 5 p.m. (Central Time), Monday through Friday. Inside the United States, call 1-800-692-9010. Outside the United States, call 314-872-8370.

A QUICK TOUR

Welcome to *Virtual Clinical Excursions*, a virtual hospital setting in which you can work with five complex patient simulations and also learn to access and evaluate the information resources that are essential for high-quality patient care.

The virtual hospital, Red Rock Canyon Medical Center, is a teaching hospital for Canyonlands State University. Within the medical center, you will work on a medical-surgical floor with a realistic architecture as well as access information resources. The floor plan in which the patient scenarios unfold is constructed from a model of a real medical center. The medical-surgical unit has:

- Five patient rooms (Room 302, Room 303, Room 304, Room 309, Room 310)
- A Nurses' Station (Room 312)
- A Supervisor's Office (Room 301)
- Two conference rooms (Room 307, Room 308)
- A nurses' lounge (Room 306)

■ BEFORE YOU START

Make sure you have your textbook nearby when you use the *Virtual Clinical Excursions Patients' Disk*. You will want to consult topic areas in your textbook frequently while working with the CD and using this workbook.

■ SUPERVISOR'S OFFICE (ROOM 301)

Just like a real-world clinical rotation, you have to let someone know when you arrive on the hospital floor—and you have to let someone know when you leave the floor. This process is completed in the Supervisor's Office (Room 301).

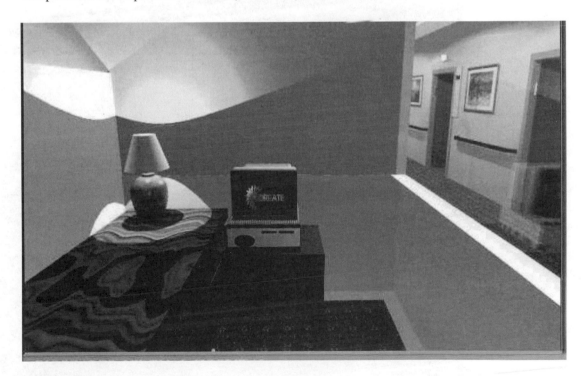

To get a 360° view of where you are "standing":

- Place the cursor in the middle of the screen.
- Hold down the mouse.
- Drag either right or left.

You will see you are in a room with an alcove to your left and a door behind you. To move into the hallway, place the cursor in the door opening and click. Once you are in the hallway, hold down the mouse and make a 360° turn.

In one direction, you will see:

- An exit sign
- An elevator
- A waiting room

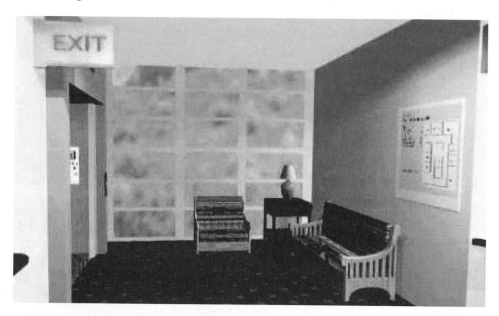

In the other direction, you will see a:

- Patient room
- Mobile computer

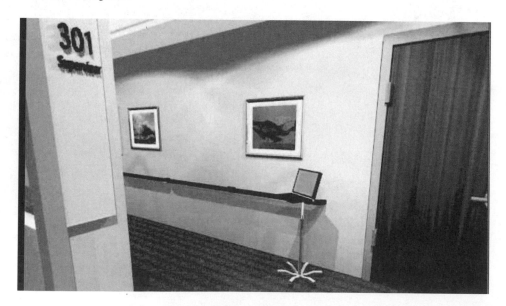

Move the cursor to a new place along the hallway outside the Supervisor's Office and click again. (Always try to place the cursor in the middle of the screen.) You should be moving along the hallway. Remember, at any point you can hold down the mouse and turn 360° in either direction. You can also hold down and move the mouse to the top or bottom of the frame, giving you views looking up or down.

■ READING ROOM

Go back into the Supervisor's Office by clicking on anything inside the room. Explore the Supervisor's Office (Room 301), and you will find another computer. This computer is a link to Canyonlands State University, the simulated university associated with the Red Rock Canyon Medical Center. Double-click on this computer, and a Web browser screen will be launched, which will open the Medical-Nursing Library in Canyonlands State University.

Click on the **Reading Room** icon, and you will see a table of icons that allows you to read short learning modules on a variety of anatomy and physiology topics.

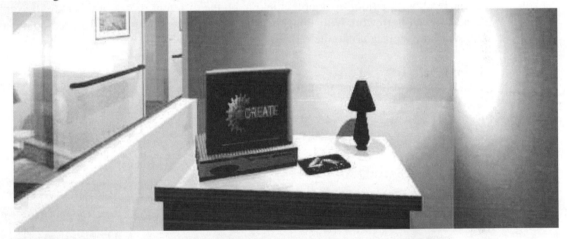

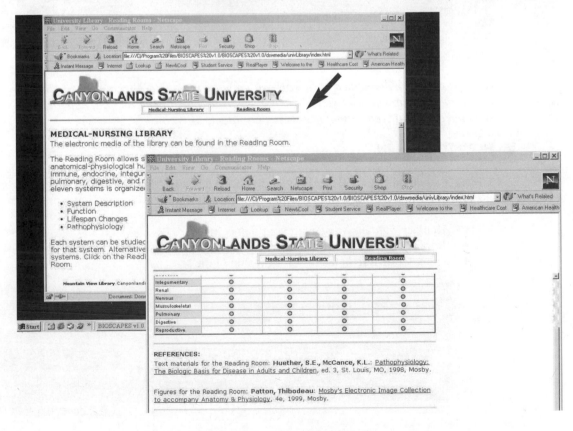

When you are ready to exit the reading room, go to the **File** icon on the browser, look at the drop-down menu, and select **Exit** or **Close**, depending on your Web browser. The browser will close, and once again you will be looking at the computer in the Supervisor's Office.

■ FLOOR MAP AND ANIMATED MAP

Move into the hallway outside the Supervisor's Office and turn right. A floor map can be found on the wall in the waiting area opposite the elevator and exit sign. To get there, click on anything in the waiting area. You should be able to see the map now, but you may not be close enough to open it. Click again on an object in the waiting area; this will move you closer. Turn to the right until you can see the map. Double-click on the map, and you will get a close-up view of the medical-surgical floor's layout. Click on the **Return** icon to exit this close-up view of the floor map.

Compare the floor map on the wall with the animated map in the upper right-hand corner of your screen. The green dot follows your position on the floor to show you where you are. You can move about the floor by double-clicking on the different rooms in this map. If you have already signed in to work with a patient, double-clicking on the patient's room on the animated map will take you right into the room.

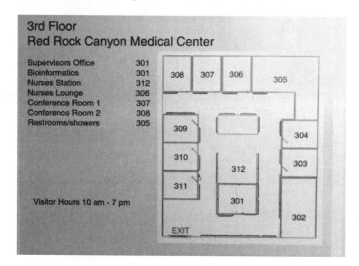
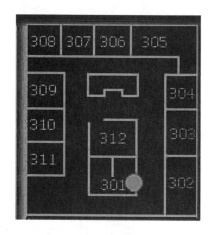

Note: If you have not signed in to work with a patient, double-clicking on a patient's room on the animated map will take you to the hallway right outside the room. If you have not yet selected a patient, you cannot access patient rooms or records.

■ HOW TO SIGN IN

To select a patient, you will need to sign in on the desktop computer in the Supervisor's Office (Room 301). Double-click on the computer screen, and a log-on screen will appear.

- Replace *Student Name* with your name.
- Replace the student ID number with your student ID number.
- Click **Continue** in the lower right side of the screen.

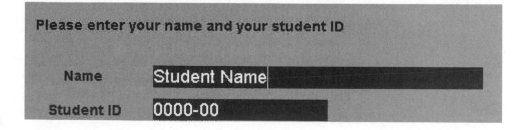

■ HOW TO SELECT A PATIENT

You can choose any one of five patients to work with. For each patient you can select either of two 4-hour shifts on Tuesday or Thursday (0700–1100 or 1100–1500). You can also select a Friday morning period in which you can review all of the data for the patient you selected. You will not, however, be able to visit patients on Friday, only review their records.

■ PATIENT LIST

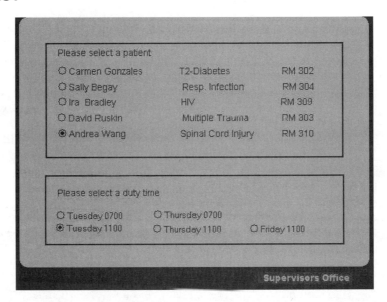

- **Carmen Gonzales (Room 302)**

  Diabetes mellitus, type 2 – An older Hispanic female with an infected leg that has become gangrenous. She has type 2 diabetes mellitus, as well as complications of congestive heart failure and osteomyelitis.

- **David Ruskin (Room 303)**

  Motor vehicle accident – A young adult African-American male admitted with a possible closed head injury and a severely fractured right humerus following a car-bicycle accident. He undergoes an open reduction and internal fixations of the right humerus.

- **Sally Begay (Room 304)**

  Respiratory infection – A Native American woman initially suspected to have a Hantavirus infection. She has a confirmed diagnosis of bacterial lung infection. This patient's complications include chronic obstructive pulmonary disease and inactive tuberculosis.

- **Ira Bradley (Room 309)**

  HIV-AIDS – A Caucasian adult male in late-stage HIV infection admitted for an opportunistic respiratory infection. He has complications of oral fungal infection, malnutrition, and wasting. Patient-family interactions also provide opportunities to explore complex psychosocial problems.

- **Andrea Wang (Room 310)**

  Spinal cord injury – A young Asian female who entered the hospital after a diving accident in which her T6 was crushed, with partial transection of the spinal cord. After a week in ICU, she has been transferred to the Medical-Surgical unit, where she is being closely monitored.

Note: You can select only one patient for one time period. If you are assigned to work with multiple patients, return to the Supervisor's Office to switch from one patient to another.

■ HOW TO FIND A PATIENT'S RECORDS

Nurses' Station (Room 312)

Within the Nurses' Station, you will see:

1. A blue notebook on the counter—this is the Medication Administration Record (MAR).
2. A bookshelf with patient charts.
3. Two desktop computers—the computer to the left of the bulletin board is used to access Red Rock Canyon Medical Center's Intranet; the computer to the right beneath the bookshelf is used to access the Electronic Patient Record (EPR). *(Note: You can also access the EPR from the mobile computer outside the Supervisor's Office, next to Room 302.)*
4. A bulletin board—this contains important information for students.

As you use these resources, you will always be able to return to the Nurses' Station (Room 312) by clicking either a **Nurses' Station** icon or a **3rd Floor** icon located next to the red cross in the lower right-hand corner of the computer screen.

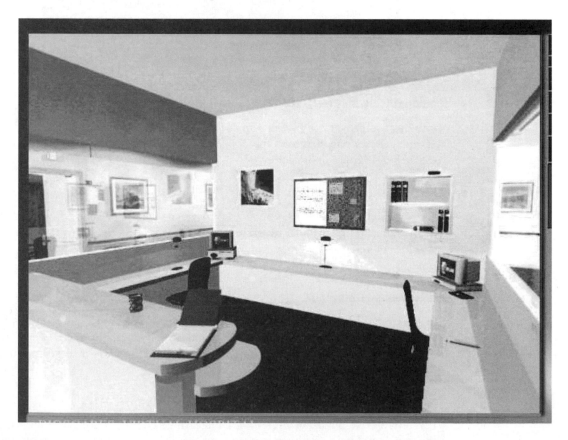

1. Medication Administration Record (MAR)

The blue notebook on the counter in the Nurses' Station (Room 312) is the Medication Administration Record (MAR), listing current 24-hour medications for each patient. Simply click on the MAR, and it opens like a notebook. Tabs allow you to select patients by room number. Each MAR sheet lists the following:

- Medications
- Route and dosage of medications
- Times of administration of medication

The MAR changes each day.

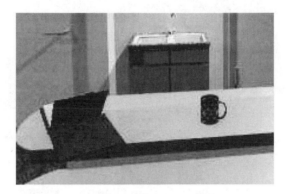

PATIENT: Gonzales, Carmen	MR# 20194873	DAY: Tuesday		
START	END	MEDICATION	2301 0700	0701 1500	1501 2300

START	END	MEDICATION	2301 / 0700	0701 / 1500	1501 / 2300
		Cefoxitin, 2 g IVPB q6h	~~0300~~ LG	~~0900~~ JS 1500	2100
		Glyburide, 3.0 mg PO qA.M., with breakfast		~~0800~~ JS	
		Blood Glucose, AC and HS 0730 = 260, 1100 = 170		~~0730~~ JS ~~1100~~ JS	
		Decrease D₅ 0.45 NS, 20 cc/hour	~~0600~~ LG		
		Morphine Sulfate, IM 2-5 mg q1-2h, PRN for severe pain 5 mg @ 0300, 0600 LG 5 mg @ 0800	~~0300~~ LG ~~0600~~ LG	~~0800~~ JS	

118%   1 of 1   8 x 14 in

302 303 **304** **309** **310**

2. Charts

In the back right-hand corner of the Nurses' Station (Room 312) is a bookshelf with patient charts. To open a chart:

- Double-click on the bookshelf.
- Click once on the chart of your choice.

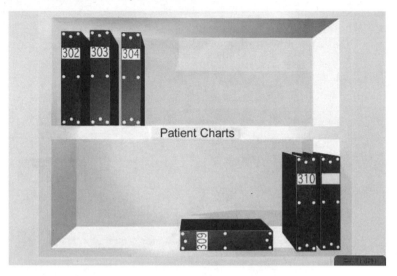

Tabs at the bottom of each patient's chart allow you to review the following data:

- Physical & History*
- Physicians' Notes
- Physicians' Orders
- Nurses' Notes
- Diagnostics Reports

- Expired MARs
- Health Team Reports
- Surgeons' Notes
- Other Reports

"Flip" forward by selecting a tab or backward by clicking on the small chart icon in the lower right side of your screen. (**Flip Back** appears on this icon once you have moved beyond the first tab.) As in the real world, the data in each patient's chart changes daily.

Note: Physical & History is a seven-page PDF file for Carmen Gonzales, David Ruskin, and Ira Bradley. Physical & History is a five-page PDF file for Andrea Wang and Sally Begay. Remember to scroll down to read all pages.

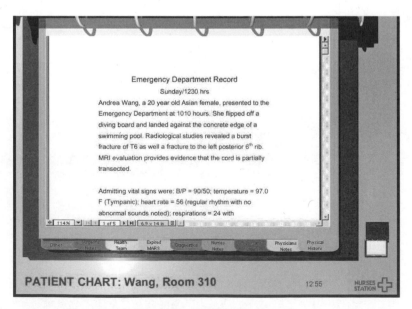

3. Two Computers

◆   **Electronic Patient Record (EPR)**

You can only access an Electronic Patient Record (EPR) once you have signed in and selected the patient in the Supervisor's Office (Room 301). The EPR can be accessed from two computers:

- Desktop computer under the bookshelf in the Nurses' Station (Room 312)
- Mobile computer outside the Supervisor's Office, next to Room 302

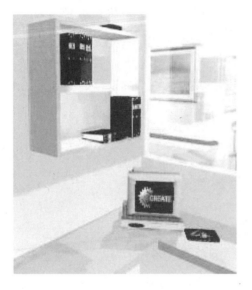
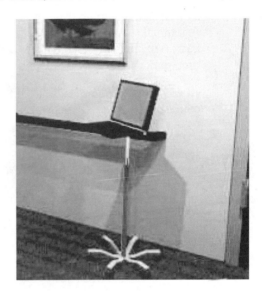

To access a patient's EPR:

- Double-click on the computer screen.
- Type in the password—it will always be **rn2b**.
- Click on **Access Records**.
- Click on the patient's name, then on **Access EPR** (or simply double-click on the patient's name).

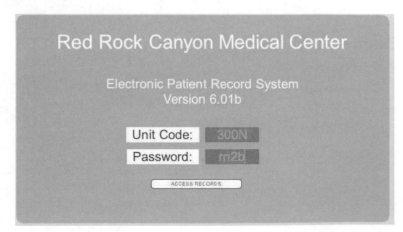

*Note: Do **not** press the Return/Enter key. If you make a mistake, simply delete the password, reenter it, and click **Access Records**. You will then enter the records system, where you find a list of patients.*

The EPR form represents a composite of commercial versions being used in hospitals and clinics. You can access the EPR:

- For a patient
- To review existing data
- To enter data you collect while working with a patient

The EPR is updated daily, so no matter what day or part of a shift you are working, there will be a current EPR with the patient's data from the past days of the current hospital stay. This type of simulated EPR allows you to examine how data for different attributes have changed over time, as well as to examine data for all of a patient's attributes at a particular time. The EPR is fully functional (as it is in a real-life hospital or clinic). You can enter such data as blood pressure, heart rate, and temperature. The EPR will not, however, allow you to enter data for a previous time period.

At the lower left corner of the EPR, there are nine icons that allow you to view different types of patient data:

- Assessment
- Admissions
- Urinanalysis
- Vital Signs
- ADL

- Blood Gases
- I&O
- Chemistry
- Hematology

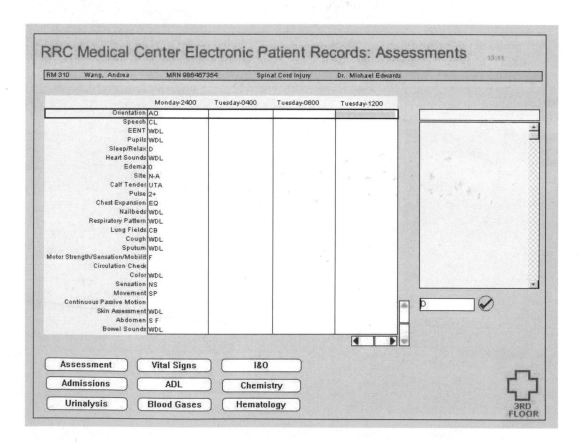

Remember, each hospital or clinic selects its own codes. The codes in the Red Rock Canyon Medical Center may be different from ones you have seen in clinical rotations that have computerized patient records.

You use the codes for the data type, selecting the code to describe your assessment findings and typing that code in the box in the lower right side of the screen, to the left of the checkmark symbol (✓).

Once the data are typed in this box, they are entered into the patient's record by clicking on the checkmark (✓). Make sure you are in the correct cell by looking for the placement of the blue box in the table. That box identifies which cell the database is "looking" at for any given moment.

You can leave the EPR by clicking on the **3rd Floor** icon in the lower right corner. This takes you back into the Nurses' Station (Room 312).

◆ Intranet

The computer on the left of the bulletin board in the Nurses' Station (Room 312) is dedicated to Red Rock Canyon Medical Center's **Intranet**. This system contains resources related to working within the hospital. Again, a double click on the screen will activate the computer. A Web browser will come up with four options (Hospital News, Employment, InfoStat, and Home). Navigate within the Intranet just as you would within a Web-based Internet site. Click on **Hospital News** and read some of the articles. The Employment icon opens a screen with descriptions of jobs available in the hospital. The InfoStat icon will connect the hospital Intranet to the Internet. *(Note: This option searches for your Internet connection, activates that connection, and takes you to the publisher's Website for your textbook.)* When in doubt, click on **Home**, which will take you back to the home page for the site.

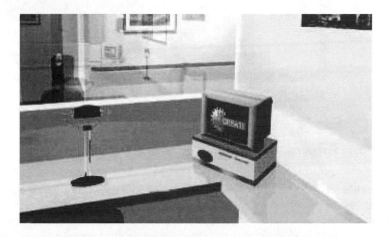

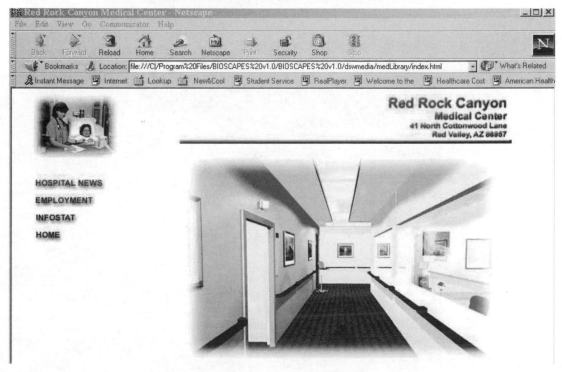

To return to the **Nurses' Station (Room 312)**, exit from the browser. This computer simulates being in a Web environment, so you have to exit from the Intranet by exiting from the browser. Click on **File**, then on **Exit** or **Close** (depending on your browser).

4. Bulletin Board

The bulletin board in the Nurses' Station (Room 312) has important information for students. Click on the board and you can read where reports are being given for patients and where the health team meetings are being held. Lessons in your workbook will direct you to these meetings and reports. Click on **Return** to exit this close-up view of the board.

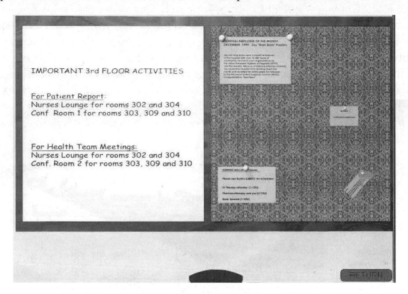

■ VISITING A PATIENT

First, go the Supervisor's Office and sign in to work with Andrea Wang for Tuesday at 0700. Now go to her room. *(Note: The quickest way to get to a patient's room is by double-clicking the room number on the animated map. You can also choose to move through the hallway until you reach the patient's door; then click on the doorknob.)* Once you are inside the room, you will see a still frame of your patient. Below this frame, you will find four icons:

- Vital Signs
- Health History
- Physical
- Medications

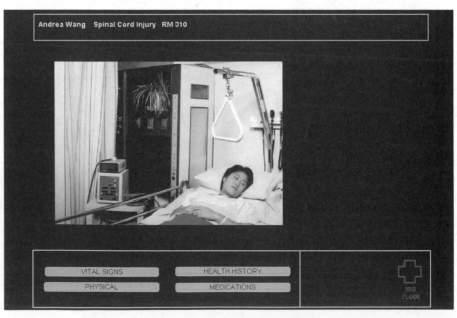

Each of these icons provides the opportunity to assess the patient or the patient's medications. When you click on an icon, you will follow a nurse through the process of collecting assessment data. The nurse will not speak to you but will rely on you to collect the data obtained during patient assessment, to record patient data in the EPR, and sometimes to make decisions after a nurse-patient interaction.

◆ **Vital Signs**

Click on **Vital Signs**; six new icons appear. Each of these new icons allows you to collect data for a particular vital sign. *(Note: You can also see two icons in the right corner.* **Continue Working with Patient** *takes you back to the main menu for this patient. Clicking on* **3rd Floor** *will take you back into the hallway.)* Click on the **Temperature** icon. You will see the nurse take the patient's temperature with a tympanic thermometer. At the end of the measurement, the temperature is shown in the animation of the thermometer to the right of the video screen. These types of interactions allow you to collect data during patient visits.

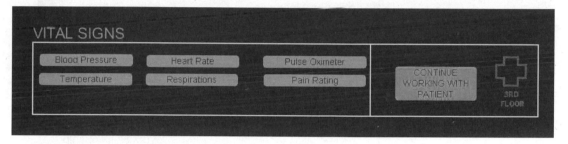

◆ **Physical Examination**

Click **Continue Working with Patient** to return to the main patient menu. Now click the **Physical** icon. Note the different areas of physical examination you can conduct. Try one.

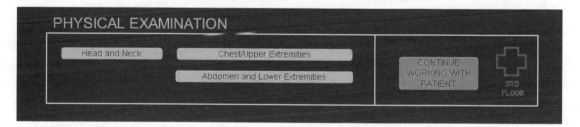

◆ **Health History**

Next, click **Continue Working with Patient** and select the **Health History** icon. In this interactive learning arena, you can ask the patient about her health history. Questions are organized into 12 categories, each of which is accessed by an icon below the video screen. Click on **Culture**, and three new icons appear in the frame to the right of the video. Click on the **Preferred Language** icon, and you will discover the language this patient prefers to use. For each of the 12 question areas, there are three topics you can explore. Thus, there are 36 different question areas related to the health history of each patient.

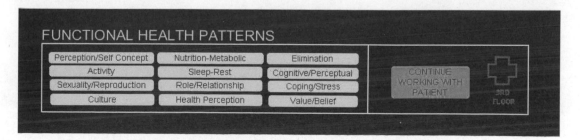

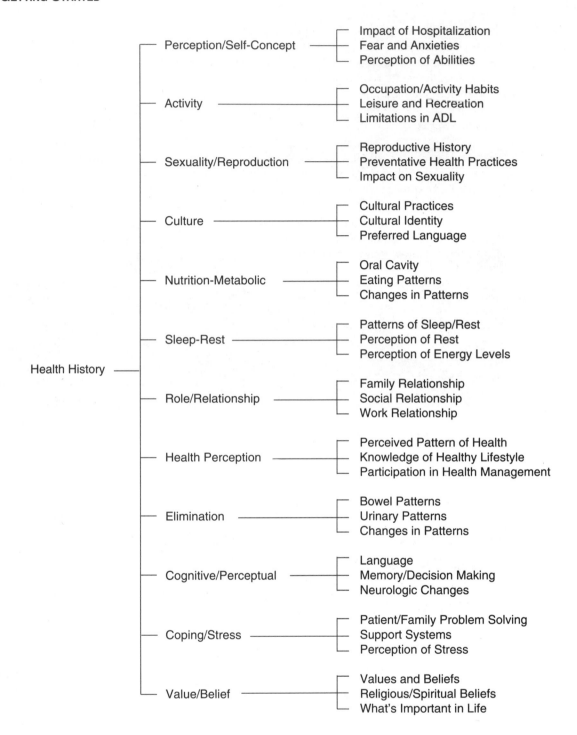

◆   **Medications**

Click **Continue Working with Patient**, and then click the **Medications** icon. Notice that you have three options within this learning environment: Review Medications, Administer, and Hold Medications. Don't click on these now, because you will need to look at this patient's records before you decide whether or not to give medications.

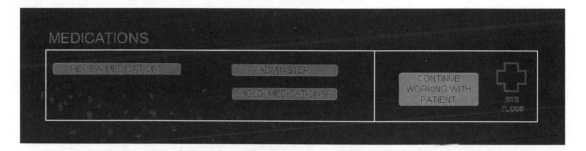

■ HOW TO QUIT OR CHANGE PATIENTS

How to Quit: If necessary, click either the **3rd Floor** icon or the **Nurses' Station** icon (depending on which screen you are currently using) to return to the medical-surgical floor. Then click on the **Quit** icon in the lower right corner of your screen.

How to Change Patients or Shifts: Go to the Supervisor's Office and double-click on the sign-in computer. Click the **Reset** icon. When the next screen appears, select a new patient or a different shift with the same patient.

A DETAILED TOUR

If you wish to understand the capabilities of the virtual hospital, take a detailed tour by going through the following section.

■ WORKING WITH A PATIENT

Sign in and select Carmen Gonzales as your patient for Tuesday at 0700 hours.

To become more familiar with the *Virtual Clinical Excursions Patients' Disk,* try the following exercises. These activities are designed to introduce you to all of the different components and learning opportunities available within the software. Each exercise will ask you to collect data on a patient.

■ REPORT

In hospitals, when one nurse's shift ends and another begins, the outgoing nurse who attended a patient will give a verbal and sometimes a written summary of that patient's condition to the incoming nurse who will assume care for the patient. This summary is called a *report* and is an important source of data to provide an overview of a patient.

Your first task is to get the report on Carmen Gonzales. Go to the bulletin board in the Nurses' Station. Double-click on the board and check the location where the attending nurse from the previous shift will give you report on this patient. Remember, Carmen Gonzales is in Room 302, so look for that room number on the bulletin board. You will find that the report is being given in the Nurses' Lounge (Room 306). Click **Return** to leave this close-up view of the bulletin board. *(Note: You can also find out where reports are being given by moving your cursor across the animated map.)* Go to Room 306 by double-clicking on the animated map. Once inside the room, click on **Report** and then on **Gonzales**. Listen to report and make a list of this patient's problems and high-priority concerns. When you are finished, click on the **3rd Floor** icon to return to the Nurses' Station.

Problems/Concerns

■ CHARTS

Find the patient charts in the bookshelf to the right of the bulletin board. Double-click on the bookshelf and find Carmen Gonzales' chart (the one labeled **302**). Click on her chart and read the section called Physical & History, including the Emergency Department Record. Determine from this information why Carmen Gonzales has been admitted to the hospital. In the space below, write a brief summary of why this patient was admitted.

■ MEDICATIONS

Open the Medication Administration Record (MAR) by clicking on the blue notebook on the counter of the Nurses' Station. Find the list of medications prescribed for Carmen Gonzales, and write down the medications that need to be given during the time period 0730–0930. For each medication, note dosage, route, and time in the chart below.

Time	Medication	Dosage	Route

Close the MAR and go inside Carmen Gonzales' room (302). Click on the **Medications** icon. You will be responsible for administering the medications ordered during the time period 0730–0930.

To become familiar with the medication options, look at the frame below the video screen. There you will find three opportunities:

- Review Medications
- Administer
- Hold Medications

Click on **Review Medications**. This brings up a frame to the right of the video screen with a list of the medications ordered for the period 0730–0930 hours. Decide whether these medications match what appears within the **Medication Administration Record (MAR)** for this time period. If they do match, you can click the **Administer** icon. If they do not match, you should select **Hold Medications**. When you are finished, click **Continue Working With Patient** to return to the patient care menu.

■ VITAL SIGNS

Vital signs are often considered the traditional signs of life and include body temperature, heart rate, respiratory rate, blood pressure, oxygen saturation of the blood, and the patient's experience of pain.

Inside Carmen Gonzales' room, click on the **Vital Signs** icon. This icon activates a pathway that allows you to measure the patient's vital signs. When you enter this pathway, you will see a short video in which the nurse informs the patient what is about to happen. Six vital signs options appear at the bottom of the screen. Each icon activates a video clip in which the respective vital sign is measured. Relevant vital signs data become available in these videos. For example, click on **Heart Rate**, and a video clip and animation of a radial pulse appear. You can measure the heart rate by counting the animated pulses during a prescribed time.

Try each of the different vital signs options to see what kinds of data are obtained. The vital signs data change over time to reflect the temporal changes you would find in a patient similar to Carmen Gonzales. You will see this most clearly if you "leave" the Tuesday time period you are currently within and "come back" on Thursday. However, you will also find changes throughout any given day (for example, differences between the 0700–1100 and 1100–1500 shifts).

Collect vital signs data for Carmen Gonzales and enter them into the following table. Note the time at which you collected these data.

Vital Signs	Findings/Time
Blood Pressure	
O$_2$ Saturation	
Heart Rate	
Respiratory Rate	
Temperature	
Pain Rating	

After you are done, click on the **3rd Floor** icon in the lower right portion of your screen. This will take you back into the hallway. Move along the hallway (or use the animated map in the upper right corner of your screen) to return to the Nurses' Station. Enter the station, and click on the computer that accesses the Electronic Patient Record (EPR). First you will see the Electronic Patient Record System entry screen. Type in **rn2b** for the password (remember, do *not* press the Return/Enter key). Then click **Access Records**, and you will see a new screen with patients listed. Click on **Carmen Gonzales** and then on **Access EPR**. Now you are in the EPR system. Click on **Vital Signs**, which will open the screen with vital signs data. Use the blue and orange arrows in the lower right-hand corner of the data table to move around within the database. Look at the data collected earlier for each of the vital signs you measured. Use these data to establish a baseline for each of the vital signs.

a. Are any of the data you collected significantly different from the baselines for those vital signs?	Circle One: Yes No
b. If "Yes," which data are different?	

■ PHYSICAL ASSESSMENT

After examining the EPR for vital signs, click the **Assessment** icon and review Carmen Gonzales' data in this area. Once you have reviewed the data and noted any areas of concern to you, close the EPR, enter Carmen Gonzales' room, and click on the **Physical** icon. This will activate the following three options for conducting a physical assessment of the patient:

- Head and Neck
- Chest/Upper Extremities
- Abdomen and Lower Extremities

Click on the **Head and Neck** icon. You will see the nurse conduct an assessment of the head and neck. At the end of the video, a series of icons appear in a frame to the right of the video screen. These icons list the different areas of the head and neck that were examined and the data obtained during the examination. The icons allow you to replay that section of the video in which the particular area was examined.

For example, if you click on **Oculomotor** (the finding is "Oculomotor function intact"), you will see a replay of the assessment of oculomotor function. Each of the icons activates only that portion of the head and neck assessment focused on the particular area described by the icon. The intention is to help you correlate each part of a physical assessment with the data obtained from that assessment—and to give you the opportunity to have the whole assessment of a region conducted beginning to end so that you can learn the process as well as its component parts. Click **Continue Working with Patient** and explore the Chest/Upper Extremities and the Abdomen and Lower Extremities options. For each area, browse through the icons that provide data on a particular area of the assessment. *(Note: The data for certain attributes found during physical assessments change for some patients as you follow them through the virtual week.)*

Focus on the examination of the abdomen and lower extremities by clicking on the option. Pay close attention to the leg wound. In the following table, record the data collected by the nurse during the examination.

Area of Examination	Findings
Abdomen	
Legs	

After you have completed the physical examination of the abdomen and lower extremities, click **Continue Working with Patient** to return to the patient care menu. From there, click on the **3rd Floor** icon and return to the Nurses' Station. Enter the data you collected in Carmen Gonzales' EPR. Compare the data that were already in the record with the data you just collected.

a. Are any of the data you collected significantly different from the baselines for those vital signs?	Circle One: Yes No
b. If "Yes," which data are different?	

■ HEALTH HISTORY

Conduct part of a health history of Carmen Gonzales. Return to her room and click on the **Health History** icon. Twelve health history areas become visible as icons below the video screen. For example, you can see Perception/Self-Concept, Activity, Sexuality/Reproduction, and so on. Note that this patient speaks Spanish and that the nurse has brought in a translator. All of the health history conversations with Carmen Gonzales are completed through translation. Clicking on any of the 12 health history icons reveals three question areas for that category. For example, if you click **Perception/Self-Concept**, a box appears to the right of the video screen with three question areas:

- Impact of Hospitalization
- Fear and Anxieties
- Perception of Abilities

Each of these three areas can be activated by clicking on their respective icons. When an icon is clicked, you will see a video in which your preceptor asks a question in the respective area and the patient answers through the translator.

Since there are 12 health history areas, with three areas of questioning for each, you have access to a total of 36 video clips that provide an opportunity to learn quite a bit about Carmen Gonzales. The questions and responses were chosen for reasons. In fact, conducting an actual health history would not unfold in such discrete and isolated moments; in the real world you would need to follow up some responses with additional questions. Other lessons in this workbook will encourage you to look at each of the health history areas and decide what additional questions need to be asked.

Unlike the vital signs and physical examination findings, the health history data do not change. The developers of *Virtual Clinical Excursions* realized that the number of videos (and the space required for storage) would become too large for the type of educational package we envisioned. We therefore decided to produce only one set of health history data-collecting opportunities. In truth, the health history would probably not change much over a week. Lessons in your workbook may have you collect health history data on the first day of care, or some of the health history queries may be assigned for Tuesday and the others for Thursday.

We recommend that you explore the health history of Carmen Gonzales by choosing some of the 12 categories and asking one or two of the three questions available for each area. When you are done exploring the health history options, leave the patient's room and go to one of the computers that allow you to access the EPR. Browse through the different data fields to see where you would enter data from the health history questions.

Remember: When you are ready to stop working with your *Virtual Clinical Excursions Patients' Disk*, click on the **Quit** icon found in the lower right-hand corner of any of the 3rd floor screens.

■ COLLECTING AND EVALUATING DATA

Each of the patient care activities generates a great deal of assessment data. Remember that after you collect data, you can go to the Nurses' Station or the mobile computer outside Room 302 and enter the data into the EPR. You also can review the data in the EPR, as well as review a patient's chart and MAR. You will get plenty of practice collecting and then evaluating data in the context of the patient's course during previous shifts.

Now, here's an important question for you:

> Did the previous sequence of exercises provide the most efficient way to assess Carmen Gonzales?

For example, you went to the patient's room to get vital signs, then back to the EPR to enter data and compare your finding with extant data. Then, you went back to the patient's room to do a physical examination, and again back to the EPR to enter and review data. If this back-and-forth process of data collection and recording seemed inefficient, remember the following:

- You want to plan all of your nursing activities to maximize efficiency while at the same time optimizing quality of patient care.
- You collect a tremendous amount of data when you work with a patient. Very few people can accurately remember all these data for more than a few minutes. Develop efficient assessment skills, and enter assessment data as soon as possible after collecting them.
- Assessment data are only the starting point for the nursing process.

Make a clear distinction between these first exercises and how you actually provide nursing care. These initial exercises were designed to involve you actively in the use of different software components. This workbook focuses on sensible practices for implementing the nursing process in ways that ensure the highest quality care of patients.

Most importantly, remember that a human being changes through time—and that these changes include both the physical and psychosocial facets of a person as a living organism. Think about this for a moment. Some patients may change physically in a very short time (a patient with emerging myocardial infarction) or more slowly (a patient with chronic illness). Patients' overall physical and psychosocial conditions may improve or deteriorate. They may have effective coping skills and familial support or feel they are alone and full of despair. In fact, each individual is a complex mix of physical and psychosocial elements, and at least some of these elements usually change through time.

Thus it is crucial *not* to think of the nursing process as a simple one-time, five-step procedure:

- Assessment
- Nursing Diagnosis
- Planning
- Implementation
- Evaluation

Rather, it is a creative and systematic approach to delivering nursing care. Furthermore, because all living organisms are constantly changing, we must apply the nursing process over and over. Each time we follow the nursing process for an individual patient, we refine our understanding of that patient's physical and psychosocial conditions based on collection and analyses of many different types of data. *Virtual Clinical Excursions* will help you develop both the creativity and the systematic approach needed to become a nurse who can deliver the highest quality care to all patients.

The following icons are used throughout the workbook to help you quickly identify particular activities and assignments:

 Indicates a reading assignment—tells you which textbook chapter(s) you should read before starting each lesson

 Indicates a writing activity

 Marks the beginning of an interactive CD-ROM activity—signals you to open or return to your *Virtual Clinical Excursions Patients' Disk*

 Indicates additional CD-ROM instructions

 Indicates questions and activities that require you to consult your textbook

LESSON **1**

The Continuum of Patient Care

 Reading Assignment: Community-Based Nursing and Home Health Care (Chapter 2)
Patients: Sally Begay, Room 304
Ira Bradley, Room 309
Andrea Wang, Room 310

In this lesson we will compare the hospital admissions and discharges of three different patients from the framework of the care continuum and from a discharge needs standpoint. Before you begin, consider the content presented in your textbook regarding continuum of care. Three phases along the continuum are presented: acute care settings, transitional care settings, and home care settings.

Review in your textbook the various types of nursing care units that are typically associated with *acute* care settings. Match each of the following terms with the corresponding description.

 Writing Activity

Description	Term
1. _____ These types of units are for patients who require frequent monitoring and more intensive care than those in a general nursing unit but are not in need of critical care placement.	a. Acute care settings
	b. Critical care
	c. Observation units
2. _____ Patients admitted to these units typically have an acute episode of a chronic medical condition, or they require care for a new condition but are not in need of advanced monitoring or supportive care.	d. General nursing units
3. _____ Care in this type of unit is provided to patients who typically have multiple complex physiologic needs, severe illness, or trauma. Care is highly focused, often involving life-supportive care and hemodynamic monitoring.	
4. _____ This term refers to care provided to acutely ill patients who are unable to care for themselves at home. These patients' needs require that they receive specialized medical and nursing care within a hospital setting.	

CD-ROM Activity

You will now conduct a brief medical record review of three patients: Sally Begay, Ira Bradley, and Andrea Wang. Open your *Virtual Clinical Excursions Patients' Disk*. First, go to the Supervisor's Office and sign in to work with Sally Begay on Thursday at 1100. Next, go to the Nurses' Station and find Sally Begay's chart. Click on the chart to open it.

- Read the entire Physical & History. (Remember to scroll down to read all pages.)
- Click on **Physicians' Orders**. Read the initial admission orders on Saturday at 1230. Note where the patient was admitted. When you are finished, click on the **Nurses' Station** icon to close the chart.

Student Notes

Go back to the Supervisor's Office. This time, sign in to work with Ira Bradley on Thursday at 1100. Next, go to the Nurses' Station and open his chart.

- Read the entire Physical & History, including the Emergency Department Report.
- Click on **Physicians' Orders**. Read the initial admission orders for Sunday at 2255. Note where the patient was admitted. When you are through, close the chart.

Student Notes

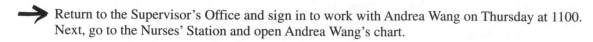 Return to the Supervisor's Office and sign in to work with Andrea Wang on Thursday at 1100. Next, go to the Nurses' Station and open Andrea Wang's chart.

- Read the entire Physical & History, including the Emergency Department Record.
- Click on **Health Team** and read the notes provided by the nurse case manager, Sara Terney. Note where the patient was originally admitted. When you are through, close the chart.

Student Notes

Answer the following questions based on what you found from your chart review.

5. Which patient was admitted to the critical care unit? (Circle one.)

   Sally Begay   Ira Bradley   Andrea Wang

6. Consider the description of critical care units in the matching activity on page 29. What data did you find in the admission orders and the Physical & History that justify this patient's admission to a critical care unit?

7. Which patient was admitted to the observation unit (telemetry)? (Circle one.)

   Sally Begay   Ira Bradley   Andrea Wang

8. Consider the description of observation units in the matching activity on page 29. What data exist in the admission orders and the Physical & History that justify this patient's admission to this type of unit?

9. Which patient was admitted to a general nursing unit? (Circle one.)

   Sally Begay   Ira Bradley   Andrea Wang

10. Consider the description of general nursing units in the matching activity on page 29. What data exist in the admission orders and the Physical & History that justify this patient's admission to this type of unit?

 Next, consider the content presented in your textbook regarding transitional care settings, long-term care settings, and home care settings. Specifically, review the terms *transitional care*, *long-term care*, and *home care*.

 11. Write a brief description of each of the following terms based on what you have read in your textbook.

Transitional care settings:

• Sub-acute care:

- Acute rehabilitation care:

Long-term care settings:

Home health care settings:

- Hospice care:

➡ Now consider the discharge needs of the three patients. First, go to the Supervisor's Office and sign in to work with Sally Begay on Thursday at 1100. Next, go to the Nurses' Station and open her chart.

- Click on **Health Team** and read the reports of the nurse case manager, the clinical nurse specialist, and the social worker. As you read, keep in mind possible discharge needs.

12. Based on what you have read in the health team report, which of the following—if ordered upon discharge from the acute care setting—would most likely benefit Sally Begay?

___ Subacute care

___ Acute rehabilitation care

___ Home care

___ Hospice care

13. In what way does Sally Begay fit the criteria for this need, based on what you identified from the description in the textbook?

➡ Go back to the Supervisor's Office and sign in to work with Ira Bradley on Thursday at 1100. Next, go to the Nurses' Station and open his chart.

- Click on **Health Team** and read the reports of the nurse case manager, the clinical nurse specialist, and the social worker. As you read, keep in mind possible discharge needs.

14. Based on what you have read in the health team report, which of the following—if ordered upon discharge from the acute care setting—would most likely benefit Ira Bradley?

___ Subacute care

___ Acute rehabilitation care

___ Home care

___ Hospice care

15. In what way does Ira Bradley fit the criteria for this need, based on what you identified from the description in the textbook?

→ Go back to the Supervisor's Office and sign in to work with Andrea Wang on Thursday afternoon. Next, go to the Nurses' Station and open her chart.

   • Click on **Health Team** and read the reports of the nurse case manager, the clinical nurse specialist, and the social worker. As you read, keep in mind possible discharge needs.

16. Based on what you have read in the health team report, which type of nursing care is being planned for Andrea Wang upon discharge from the acute care setting?

___ Subacute care

___ Acute rehabilitation care

___ Home care

___ Hospice care

17. In what way does Andrea Wang fit the criteria for this need, based on what you identified from the description in the textbook?

18. Read the discussion of case management in the textbook. What does the term *case management* mean?

Overview

19. Consider any or all of the health team reports you read. How does the health team report of the nurse case manager differ from the clinical specialist's report and the social worker's report? Compare and contrast the differences among the three reports.

Focus of the Nurse Case Manager

Focus of the Clinical Nurse Specialist

Focus of the Social Worker

Adult Development

 Reading Assignment: Adult Development (Chapter 3)
Patients: Andrea Wang, Room 310
David Ruskin, Room 303

Adults work through many developmental stages. Although the textbook presents several theories of adult development, you will note many similarities. For this lesson, we will analyze and compare the developmental stages of the five patients in Red Rock Canyon Medical Center.

 1. Begin this activity by reviewing some of the general concepts presented in your textbook regarding the three age classifications—young adulthood, middle adulthood, and older adulthood. Fill in some of the expected developmental tasks for each of the following age classifications.

Writing Activity

Classification	Expected Developmental Tasks
Young Adulthood	

Classification	Expected Developmental Tasks
Middle Adulthood	
Older Adulthood	

CD-ROM Activity

Now that you have reviewed the various age classifications, you will apply these concepts to each of the patients in Red Rock Canyon Medical Center.

2. Fill in the following table with each patient's biologic age and the developmental stage (young adulthood, middle adulthood, and older adulthood) you would anticipate based on the age. To find the patient's age, go to the Supervisor's Office and sign in on Tuesday at 0700 for the patient. Next, find the Electronic Patient Record (EPR). You can access the EPR from two computers: the desktop computer under the bookshelf in the Nurses' Station or the mobile computer outside the Supervisor's Office, next to Room 302. Click on the computer, enter the password, and click **Access Records.** Click on the patient's name and **Access EPR** to open the EPR (or simply double-click the patient's name). Click on **Admissions** and find the patient's age in the Admissions Profile. (You will have to repeat these steps for each patient.)

Name	Age	Developmental Stage (based on age)
Carmen Gonzales		
Sally Begay		
Ira Bradley		
David Ruskin		
Andrea Wang		

Health care workers often make assumptions about their patients based on age. It is important to consider that there is a great deal of variability in developmental stages of adults. Assessment of developmental stage and related concerns should be explored with all patients.

3. Place an **X** next to all of the following factors that you think play a role in adult development.

___ Age   ___ Activity level

___ Culture   ___ Independence

___ General health   ___ Family interactions

___ Living arrangement   ___ Self-concept and self-esteem

Complete an adult developmental assessment on Andrea Wang. First, go to the Supervisor's Office and sign in to work with Andrea Wang for the 0700 shift on Tuesday. Then go into her room and click on **Health History**. Collect data by asking the patient about various areas of the functional health patterns. Compare data you collect with the typical tasks you would expect someone her age to be engaged in.

4. In what way is Andrea Wang consistent with the typical 20-year-old? What sorts of issues does she face that are not consistent with those of the typical 20-year-old? Record your findings below.

Consistent Tasks	**Inconsistent Tasks or Concerns**

Complete an adult developmental assessment on David Ruskin. First, go to the Supervisor's Office and sign in to work with David Ruskin for the 0700 shift on Tuesday. Then go to his room and click on **Health History**. Collect data by asking the patient about various areas of the functional health patterns. Compare data you collect with the typical tasks you would expect someone his age to be engaged in.

5. In what ways is David Ruskin consistent with the typical 31-year-old? What sorts of issues does he face that are not consistent with those of the typical 31-year-old? Record your findings below.

Consistent Tasks   **Inconsistent Tasks or Concerns**

6. Now that you have completed a developmental assessment on Andrea Wang and David Ruskin, compare your findings. What similarities do they share? What differences did you find? How can the nurse use this information to provide care and education for both of these patients?

LESSON 3

Health History and Physical Examination— Part I

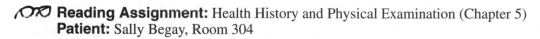 **Reading Assignment:** Health History and Physical Examination (Chapter 5)
Patient: Sally Begay, Room 304

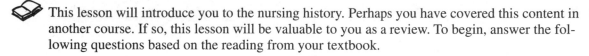 This lesson will introduce you to the nursing history. Perhaps you have covered this content in another course. If so, this lesson will be valuable to you as a review. To begin, answer the following questions based on the reading from your textbook.

Writing Activity

1. What is the primary purpose of conducting a nursing history and physical examination?

2. How does a medical history differ from a nursing history?

3. What is the difference between subjective data and objective data?

4. What are the various sources of subjective data for a given patient?

The nursing history presented in the textbook is based on functional health patterns. Match each of the following descriptions or types of data with the corresponding functional health pattern. Refer to your textbook for help. (Answers may be used more than once.)

Description or Type of Data	Functional Health Pattern
5. _____ Identification of current stresses	a. Health Perception/ Health Management
6. _____ Focus on personal relationships	
7. _____ Body image and self-description	b. Nutrition/Metabolic
8. _____ Spiritual or religious preferences	c. Elimination
9. _____ Capacity to learn; how patient learns best	d. Activity/Exercise
10. _____ Practice of health habits and ways the patient stays healthy	e. Sleep/Rest
11. _____ Energy needed to carry out daily activities.	f. Cognitive/Perceptual
12. _____ Onset of menarche or menopause	g. Self-Perception/ Self-Concept
13. _____ Family history	
14. _____ Condition of skin and ability for wounds to heal	h. Role/Relationship
15. _____ Questions related to the ability to see and hear	i. Sexuality/Reproductive
16. _____ Identification of known risk factors for disease	j. Coping/Stress Tolerance
17. _____ Questions regarding recent losses or changes	k. Value/Belief
18. _____ Pattern of urinary and bowel elimination	
19. _____ Personal role or roles in life	
20. _____ Questions regarding ability to perform activities of daily living	
21. _____ Amount of sleep and degree of rest a patient experiences	
22. _____ Questions regarding oral intake and food preferences	
23. _____ Cultural preferences or values	
24. _____ Questions regarding pain	
25. _____ Methods of contraception and facilitation of conception	
26. _____ Questions regarding adherence to prescribed therapy	
27. _____ Questions about condition of teeth and ability to chew foods	
28. _____ Patient's feelings about the worth of life and health	

CD-ROM Activity

Report to the Supervisor's Office and sign in to work with Sally Begay for Tuesday at 0700. Go to the Nurses' Station and find her chart. Open the chart and read the entire Physical & History.

29. For each heading in the left column below, describe the type of data you found in that section of Sally Begay's Physicians' History.

Physicians' History	Type of Data Included
History of present illness	
Family history	
Social history	
Medical history	

Physicians' History	Type of Data Included

Current medications

Review of systems

30. Why should a nurse review the Physicians' History?

31. Consider the data documented by the physician in Sally Begay's history. Were any data abnormal or out of the ordinary? In other words, what data suggested possible problem areas for the patient? Record your findings below.

Data from Physicians' History that are considered out of the ordinary:

32. Close Sally Begay's chart. Now go to her room and conduct a nursing history. Click on **Health History** and systematically go through all the available question areas. Record your data regarding functional health patterns below and on the next two pages.

Note to student: Keep in mind that although the nursing history used at Red Rock Canyon Medical Center is similar to the functional health patterns discussed in your textbook, you will notice some variations. Regardless of the presentation used on the CD, organize your data based on functional health patterns as presented in your textbook.

Nursing History—Functional Health Pattern Data

Health Perception/Health Promotion

Nutritional-Metabolic

Elimination

Nursing History—Functional Health Pattern Data

Activity/Exercise

Sleep-Rest

Cognitive/Perceptual

Self-Perception/Self-Concept

Nursing History—Functional Health Pattern Data

Role/Relationship

Sexuality/Reproductive

Coping/Stress

Value/Belief

33. Consider the data you recorded for question 32. What data did you find out of the ordinary (negative functioning), suggesting a problem or concern? Go back through your data and underline any data you consider to be out of the ordinary.

34. Now compare the data you recorded for question 32 with the functional health patterns history format in your textbook (Table 5-2). What additional questions do you wish the nurse would have asked?

Health History and Physical Examination— Part II

Reading Assignment: Health History and Physical Examination (Chapter 5)
Patient: Sally Begay, Room 304

This lesson focuses on the physical examination. Perhaps you have covered this content in another course. If so, this lesson will be valuable to you as a review. Begin by reviewing the types and techniques of physical examination.

 Writing Activity

1. Several types of physical examinations are listed below. For each type, write a brief description.

Type of Examination	Description
Focused examination	
Comprehensive examination	

Type of Examination	Description
Bedside or shift-to-shift examination	

2. Several techniques used during physical examination are listed below and on the next page. For each technique, write a brief description. Refer to your textbook if necessary.

Technique	Description of Technique
Inspection	
Palpation	
Percussion	

Auscultation

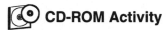

CD-ROM Activity

Report to the Supervisor's Office and sign in to work with Sally Begay for the Tuesday 0700 shift. Go to the Nurses' Station and find her chart. Open the chart and browse through the Physical & History.

3. Read the section titled Physical. Referring to the following list of headings, describe the type of data you found in each section of the physical examination.

Physical Examination	Type of Data Included
HEENT	
Cardiopulmonary	
Neurologic	

Physical Examination	Type of Data Included
Musculoskeletal	
Gastrointestinal	
Genitourinary	

4. Consider the data documented by the physician in Sally Begay's physical examination. Were any data abnormal or out of the ordinary? In other words, what data suggested possible problem areas for the patient? Record abnormal findings below.

Data from physician examination that are considered abnormal findings:

5. Based on what you have learned so far, what kinds of cultural issues might become apparent as you perform a physical examination of Sally Begay?

 6. Close Sally Begay's chart. Now go to her room (304) and conduct a physical examination. Click on **Physical** and **Vital Signs** and systematically go through all of the available examination options. As you conduct your examination, do the following three things and record your findings below and on the next two pages.

    a. Identify the examination techniques performed by the nurse on the CD.
    b. Critique the nurse on the CD. You should notice a few mistakes made in the technique used and/or the documentation done. Can you find them?
    c. Record the examination findings.

Area Assessed	What techniques did the nurse use?	What mistakes did you notice in performance or documentation?
Head and Neck		

Area Assessed	What techniques did the nurse use?	What mistakes did you notice in performance or documentation?
Chest/Upper Extremities		
Abdomen and Lower Extremities		

Documentation of Findings

Area Assessed	Findings	
Vital Signs	Temperature: _____	Oxygen saturation: _____
	Heart rate: _____	Blood pressure: _____
	Respiratory rate: _____	Pain rating: _____
Head and Neck		

Area Assessed	What techniques did the nurse use?	What mistakes did you notice in performance or documentation?
Chest/Upper Extremities		
Abdomen and Lower Extremities		

7. Are any of the nursing physical examination data you recorded considered abnormal findings? Go back through your previous findings and underline any abnormal data.

8. Consider data in the nursing history (from Lesson 3) and the nursing physical examination. What should a nurse do with this data once collected?

Patient Teaching

 Reading Assignment: Patient Teaching (Chapter 6)
Patient: Carmen Gonzales, Room 302

You have been assigned to assist with patient teaching for Carmen Gonzales. She is a 56-year-old female admitted to the hospital on Sunday evening through the Emergency Department with a diagnosis of gangrene and osteomyelitis of the left lower leg, diabetes mellitus type 2, and congestive heart failure.

 Writing Activity

1. Review the two different philosophies or frameworks for patient education presented in the textbook. Compare and contrast these approaches below and on the next page.

Patient Teaching Approach	Description
Compliance Approach	

Patient Teaching Approach	Description
Empowerment Approach	

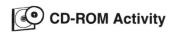 **CD-ROM Activity**

Go to the Supervisor's Office and sign in to work with Carmen Gonzales for the Thursday 1100 shift. Then go to one of the computers from which you can access the EPR. Open the EPR for Carmen Gonzales. Next, click on **Admissions** and read the Admissions Profile.

2. Identify significant data from the Admissions Profile that helps you gain an understanding of Carmen Gonzales and her needs from a teaching perspective.

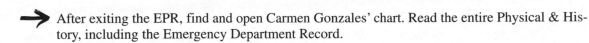

After exiting the EPR, find and open Carmen Gonzales' chart. Read the entire Physical & History, including the Emergency Department Record.

3. Identify significant data from the Emergency Department Record and other sections of the Physical & History that help you gain an understanding of Carmen Gonzales and her needs from a teaching perspective.

4. Part of developing the overall teaching plan and goals for Carmen Gonzales is dependent on her individual characteristics and her specific health care problems. The textbook identifies several variables to consider, including age, culture, educational level, self-efficacy, and psychologic state. Use your textbook to complete the following exercise.

   a. In the second column of the following table, fill in general descriptions of the patient variables listed. You will fill in the third column later.

Patient Variable	Description from Textbook	Application to Carmen Gonzales
Age		
Culture		

Patient Variable	Description from Textbook	Application to Carmen Gonzales
Educational Level		
Self-Efficacy		
Psychologic State		

b. Consider data you previously obtained from the Physicians' History and the Admissions Profile. Use the applicable data to begin filling in the third column of the table on page 59, describing how these variables apply specifically to Carmen Gonzales.

→ c. Now go to Carmen Gonzales' room. Click on **Health History** and collect data. Add any relevant data to the third column of the table.

5. Consider the communication of the nurse conducting the interview with Carmen Gonzales. What behaviors did you observe that were positive communication skills and would facilitate patient teaching?

6. Review the key question list in the following table. Using the data you just collected from the nursing health history, the Physical & History, and the Admissions Profile, indicate which of the key questions for patient teaching assessment have already been addressed. Place an **X** next to those questions where you have sufficient data. Place an **O** next to those areas where additional assessment still needs to be conducted.

Table 5-1   Assessment of Characteristics That Affect Patient Teaching

Characteristic	Key Questions
Readiness to learn	___ What has your physician or nurse practitioner told you about your health problem?
	___ What behaviors could make your problem better or worse?
Biophysical	___ What is the primary diagnosis?
	___ Are there additional diagnoses?
	___ Is the patient acutely ill?
	___ How old is the patient?
	___ What is the patient's current mental status?
	___ What is the patient's hearing ability? Visual ability? Motor ability?
	___ Is the patient fatigued? In pain?
	___ What medications is the patient on? How might these affect learning?
Psychologic	___ Does the patient appear anxious? Afraid? Depressed? Defensive?
	___ Is the patient in a state of denial?
Sociocultural	___ Does the patient have family or close friends?
	___ What is the patient's belief regarding his or her illness or treatment?
	___ Is the proposed change consistent with the patient's cultural values?
Socioeconomic	___ Does the patient work?
	___ What is the patient's occupation?
	___ What is the patient's living arrangement?
Learning style	___ Does the patient "learn best" through visual (reading), auditory (tape or lecture), or physical stimuli (demonstration)?
	___ In what kind of environment does the patient learn best? Formal classroom? Informal setting, such as home or office? Alone or among peers? What prior learning experiences were helpful?

 Go to the Nurses' Station and find the location of the health team meeting for Carmen Gonzales. Attend the meeting, listening carefully to the suggestions of the three individuals. If desired, go back to the patient's chart, click on **Health Team**, and read the written reports.

7. Below and on the following page, record some of the key issues the clinical nurse specialist, nurse case manager, and social worker have identified regarding Carmen Gonzales' discharge planning.

Discharge Planning Team Report—Student Notes

Health Team Member	Key Issues from Report
Rose Simpson, Case Manager	

Health Team Member	Key Issues from Report
Louise Johnson, CNS	
Kris Holmes, MSW	

8. Considering everything you currently know about Carmen Gonzales, make a list of *at least* five different things you could potentially teach this patient to enhance her care once she goes home.

9. Choose one of the patient teaching needs from your list in question 8. In the space below, address some of the issues that would be central to your teaching strategy.

Issue	How will you deal with this?
Communication	
Method of Teaching	
Involvement of Patient and Family	

Stress Response

 Reading Assignment: Nursing Management: Stress (Chapter 7)
Patient: David Ruskin, Room 303

This lesson focuses on the response to physical and psychologic stress. You will conduct an analysis and application of the stress response by considering the effect of stress on one of the Red Rock Canyon Medical Center patients, David Ruskin.

 Begin by reviewing the three theories of stress presented in your textbook. Match each of the following theories with the corresponding description.

/ **Writing Activity**

Stress Theory	**Description**
1. _____ Stress as a stimulus	a. A particular relationship between the person and the environment that taxes or exceeds his or her resources.
2. _____ Stress as a transaction	
3. _____ Stress as a response (general adaptation syndrome)	b. A nonspecific response of the body to any demand made on it, physical or psychologic.
	c. A stimulus that causes a response; frequent life changes make individuals more vulnerable to illness.

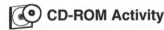 **CD-ROM Activity**

Go to the Supervisor's Office and sign in to work with David Ruskin on Tuesday at 0700. To find out what happened to this patient, go to the Nurses' Station and open his chart. Read the Physical & History, including the Emergency Department Report. Then click on **Nurses' Notes**. Read the nurses' notes for Sunday and Monday.

4. List the physical stressors David Ruskin experienced on Sunday.

73

The physiologic response to stress is initiated with the processing of the stressful stimuli by the cerebral cortex. The hypothalamus essentially triggers activation in the sympathetic nervous system, and stimulation of the anterior and posterior pituitary glands. Match each of the following physical responses with the corresponding triggering event. (Answers will be used more than once. Refer to your textbook for help if necessary.)

Physical Response	**Triggering Event**
5. _____ Increased ADH secretion	a. Stimulation of sympathetic activity
6. _____ Increased epinephrine	
7. _____ Increased blood glucose	b. Stimulation of anterior pituitary gland hormone
8. _____ Decreased peristalsis	
9. _____ Increased aldosterone secretion	c. Stimulation of posterior pituitary gland
10. _____ Decreased immune response	
11. _____ Increased cardiac output	
12. _____ Dilation of vessels in skeletal muscles	
13. _____ Decreased allergic response	
14. _____ Increased norepinephrine secretion	

15. For each of the following vital signs or body functions, indicate what you guess David Ruskin's physical reaction was during the time immediately following the accident. Mark with ↑ or ↓, unless otherwise indicated.

___ Blood pressure   ____ Gastrointestinal motility

___ Heart rate   ____ Perspiration

___ Respiratory rate   ____ Pupils (**Constriction** or **Dilation**)

16. Note David Ruskin's admitting vital signs documented in the Emergency Department. Record them in the spaces provided.

Temperature _____ Heart rate _____ Respiration _____ Blood pressure _____

17. Based on his vital signs at the time of Emergency Department evaluation, which stage would you guess David Ruskin was experiencing? (Circle the stage.)

Stage of alarm

Stage of resistance

Stage of exhaustion

18. Consider David Ruskin's condition now—Tuesday morning, 2 days post-injury. Conduct a nursing assessment of the patient's stress and his ability to cope with it. In the space below, identify current possible sources of David Ruskin's stress. Then identify factors in his life that help him resist stress (see your textbook for the seven conditioning factors). Use data from the following three sources to complete your assessment:

- Chart: Physical & History
- EPR: Admissions Profile
- Inside David Ruskin's room:
  - Click on **Health History**; collect data from the nursing history.
  - Click on **Vital Signs**, then **Pain Rating**.

Current Possible Sources of Stress	Factors That Help to Resist Stress

19. The nurse should assess not only for stressors the patient may be experiencing but also for adequate coping measures. Below is a list of coping resources discussed in the textbook. Circle all that seem to apply to David Ruskin based on the data you have collected.

Robust health	Communication skills	Self-efficacy
High energy level	Collection of information	Spiritual faith
High morale	Social networks	Adequate finances

20. Based on your assessment of David Ruskin's stressors, factors that help him resist stress, and coping measures, what specific nursing interventions can you think of that will assist this patient further in managing the stress he is currently experiencing?

 21. What is your overall evaluation of how David Ruskin is currently handling his stress? Does he seem to be managing it well? Do you have any areas of concern that could prove to be problematic? Which, if any, of the nursing diagnoses listed in Table 7-9 of your textbook are applicable to David Ruskin?

Complementary and Alternative Therapies

 Reading Assignment: Complementary and Alternative Therapies (Chapter 8)
Patients: Carmen Gonzales, Room 302
David Ruskin, Room 303
Sally Begay, Room 304
Ira Bradley, Room 309
Andrea Wang, Room 310

This lesson focuses on the possible application of various complementary and alternative therapies for the patients in Red Rock Canyon Medical Center. For this lesson, you will not need to use your *Virtual Clinical Excursions* CD.

 Before you begin, review some of the basic concepts presented in your textbook regarding complementary and alternative therapies.

Writing Activity

Indicate whether the following statements regarding complementary or alternative medicine (CAM) are true or false.

1. _____ CAM is considered overall more effective than allopathic medicine.

2. _____ Allopathic medicine is considered better for some conditions, whereas CAM may be more effective for other conditions.

3. _____ Approximately 75% of people in the United States rely on one or more forms of CAM.

4. _____ Worldwide, the United States has been the leader in the development and the acceptance of CAM.

5. _____ Many insurance companies are now covering the costs for certain types of CAM therapies.

6. What is the primary difference between complementary and alternative therapies?

Match each of the following descriptions with the corresponding complementary or alternative therapy. Use your textbook for help.

Description	CAM
7. _____ Guided or self-directed practice for relaxing the body and mind.	a. Chiropractic therapy
8. _____ Includes many techniques and methods (herbal, acupuncture, massage, Qigong, etc.)	b. Native-American practices
9. _____ Method of producing analgesia by inserting thin needles along a series of lines or channels.	c. Latin-American practices
10. _____ Use of a variety of medicinal plants for treatment of a large number of ailments, from depression to cancer.	d. Traditional Chinese practices
11. _____ The practitioner directs own interpersonal energy flow through his or her hands to help heal another person.	e. Relaxation
12. _____ Part of therapy is making contact with spirits to ask direction in bringing healing to people. Contact is made by the shaman.	f. Hypnotherapy
13. _____ Manipulation of soft tissue through stroking, rubbing, or kneading to increase circulation, improve muscle tone, and produce relaxation.	g. Guided imagery
14. _____ Concentration on an image; used to help relieve pain or discomfort.	h. Acupuncture
15. _____ Treatment involves the manipulation of the spinal column; based on theory that state of health is determined by condition of the nervous system.	i. Therapeutic touch
16. _____ Use of visual or auditory information about autonomic physiologic functions of the body through the use of instruments.	j. Biofeedback
17. _____ Induction of trance states and therapeutic suggestion; used for treatment of paralysis, headaches, addictions, and pain.	k. Massage therapy
18. _____ System that includes the use of curanderas, humoral model, and folk remedies.	l. Herbal therapy

Now consider the application of these various complementary therapies to each of the patients in Red Rock Canyon Medical Center.

19. Below and on the next four pages, you will find a brief summary of data for each patient. Based on this data, circle the complementary therapies that are most likely to be accepted by the patient and might be helpful to the patient if offered. Justify your answers in the right-hand column.

Patient Data	Complementary Therapies	Justification for or Against Use
Carmen Gonzales **Room 302** **56-year-old female** **Dx:** Diabetes mellitus type 2, CHF, osteomyelitis **Cultural group:** Hispanic-American **Primary issues:** • Having a great deal of pain in the leg from the foot infection • Has lack of understanding of medications, diet, and disease processes • Very anxious about going home and managing care • Insufficient social and financial support **Other data:** • Is Catholic—indicated an interest in having a priest visit her	Chiropractic therapy Native-American practices Latin-American practices Traditional Chinese practices Relaxation Hypnotherapy Guided imagery Acupuncture Therapeutic touch Biofeedback Massage therapy Herbal therapy	

Patient Data	Complementary Therapies	Justification for or Against Use
David Ruskin **Room 303** **31-year-old male**	Chiropractic therapy	
Dx: Bike accident—CHI and fractured humerus **Cultural:** African-American **Primary issues:** • Having a great deal of pain in the arm and headaches • Initially had some confusion from CHI • Concerns about regaining indepen-dence and athletic training schedule	Native-American practices Latin-American practices Traditional Chinese practices	
Other data: • Very interested in diet and exercise and maintaining high level of health • Describes self as spiritual, but not religious • Well-educated man—finishing master's degree • Good social and financial support	Relaxation Hypnotherapy Guided imagery Acupuncture Therapeutic touch Biofeedback Massage therapy Herbal therapy	

Patient Data	Complementary Therapies	Justification for or Against Use
Sally Begay **Room 304** **58-year-old female**	Chiropractic therapy	
Dx: Bacterial pneumonia, chronic bronchitis, hypertension **Cultural:** Traditional Navajo	Native-American practices	
Primary issues: • Has problems with shortness of breath and fatigue • Is concerned about keeping up with work on farm at home	Latin-American practices	
• Lives in rural setting miles from primary health care provider; access to health care is concern	Traditional Chinese practices	
• Lives in rural area; is in need of educational outreach to prevent further infections	Relaxation	
• Need to provide culturally sensitive care	Hypnotherapy	
	Guided imagery	
Other data: • Cultural practices important to her are medicine man and regular doctor	Acupuncture	
• Recently had healing ceremony done for her and will have another one when she gets home	Therapeutic touch	
• Good social support	Biofeedback	
	Massage therapy	
	Herbal therapy	

Patient Data	Complementary Therapies	Justification for or Against Use
Ira Bradley **Room 309** **43-year-old male**	Chiropractic therapy	
Dx: Late-stage HIV, *Pneumocystis carinii* pneumonia, candidiasis, Kaposi's sarcoma	Native-American practices	
Cultural: American Jewish **Primary issues:** • Pain/discomfort • Nutrition • Oral mucosa • Chronic fatigue	Latin-American practices	
• Depression (knows he is dying) • Ineffective family coping	Traditional Chinese practices	
• Lack of adequate financial and social support	Relaxation	
Other data: • Sees psychotherapist for depression	Hypnotherapy	
• Does not want hospital chaplain, but would appreciate visit from rabbi	Guided imagery	
	Acupuncture	
	Therapeutic touch	
	Biofeedback	
	Massage therapy	
	Herbal therapy	

Patient Data	Complementary Therapies	Justification for or Against Use
Andrea Wang **Room 310** **20-year-old female**	Chiropractic therapy	
Dx: Acute spinal cord injury; paralysis **Cultural:** Chinese-American **Primary issues:**	Native-American practices	
• Paralysis— paraplegia • Regaining independence	Latin-American practices	
• Resuming relationship with boyfriend • Sexuality • Resuming education/ career goals • Concern regarding care for parents	Traditional Chinese practices	
• Ineffective family coping	Relaxation	
• Possible lack of adequate social support	Hypnotherapy	
Other data:		
• Is a first-generation Chinese-American; primarily has Western values; however, some Chinese traditions practiced at home (mainly by parents)	Guided imagery	
	Acupuncture	
	Therapeutic touch	
	Biofeedback	
	Massage therapy	
	Herbal therapy	

20. In the previous activity, you were limited to the listed choices of complementary therapies. Now you are encouraged to consider other therapies that each of these patients might benefit from. Below, list additional complementary therapies discussed in your textbook that might be appropriate to offer to these patients.

Patient	Additional Therapies	Justification
Carmen Gonzales		
David Ruskin		
Sally Begay		
Ira Bradley		
Andrea Wang		

Pain

/oʊɔ **Reading Assignment:** Nursing Management: Pain (Chapter 9)
Patients: David Ruskin, Room 303
          Ira Bradley, Room 309

In this activity, you will compare the pain experience of two different patients—from assessment to management. To do this, you will complete a pain assessment tool on the following two patients:
- David Ruskin, a 31-year-old male patient who was hit by a car while riding his bike. This patient has many injuries, including a closed head injury, a fracture to the right arm, and a chest contusion.
- Ira Bradley, a 43-year-old male who was admitted to the hospital with late-stage HIV, *Pneumocystis carinii* pneumonia, candidiasis and Kaposi's sarcoma.

CD-ROM Activity

1. Review the pain assessment tool on the following page. Complete a pain assessment tool for David Ruskin and Ira Bradley based on data you collect from various parts of the charts as well from each patient. (*Note: you may not find all the information you need to complete the tool.*) Specifically, you should do all of the following for each patient:

- Go to the Supervisor's Office and sign in to work with the patient on Tuesday at 0700.

- Proceed to the Nurses' Station and open the patient's chart. Read the Physical & History, including the Emergency Room Report.

- Click on the **Nurses' Notes** and read the notes from Sunday until present.

- Click on **Expired MARs**. Determine the following: What pain medication has the patient received since admission? What dose has the patient received? How often has the medication been given?

- Close the chart and open the patient's EPR. Click on **Vital Signs** and review the previous pain assessment for the patient since admission.

- Close the EPR and open the MAR. What medications are available to the patient today for pain?

- Close the MAR and go into the patient's room. Click on **Vital Signs**, then **Pain Assessment**. Listen to the patient describe the pain. Click on **Continue Working with Patient**, then on **Medications** to see what medications the nurse is preparing to give. Finally, click on **Health History** and select various questions to collect data. Note any data that might be helpful in explaining the pain experience for the patient.

Pain Assessment Tool—David Ruskin
Tuesday 0800

Etiology (disease process and physical findings associated with pain) _____

_____

Type of Pain (circle one) ⟶ acute   chronic nonmalignant   malignant

Location of Pain (indicate location of pain using figure in box)

Right Left   Left Right

Description of the Pain Pattern

Pain Intensity

| 0 | 1 | 2 | 3 | 4 | 5 | 6 | 7 | 8 | 9 | 10 |

Description of the Pain Quality

Variables Affecting the Pain Experience

Affective

Behavioral

Cognitive

Record of Pain Medications Given and Effectiveness

Day	Medication, Dose, and Time Given	Effectiveness
Sunday		
Monday		
Tuesday		

Pain Assessment Tool—Ira Bradley
Tuesday 0800

Etiology (disease process and physical findings associated with pain) _____

_____

Type of Pain (circle one) ⟶ acute   chronic nonmalignant   malignant

Location of Pain (indicate location of pain using figure in box)

Right   Left   Left   Right

Description of the Pain Pattern

Pain Intensity

0 1 2 3 4 5 6 7 8 9 10

Description of the Pain Quality

Variables Affecting the Pain Experience

Affective

Behavioral

Cognitive

Record of Pain Medications Given and Effectiveness

Day	Medication, Dose, and Time Given	Effectiveness
Sunday		
Monday		
Tuesday		

2. What additional data would have been helpful to complete the pain assessment tool? In the space below, write additional questions you would have asked either patient or identify data you think should have been on the chart.

3. Compare the data on the two pain assessment tools. What similarities do you see? What differences are there?

Similarities	Differences

4. How do the terms *mild pain*, *moderate pain*, and *severe pain* correlate to the pain intensity scale?

5. How should the pain intensity scale ratings given by the two patients be interpreted? (Circle one for each patient.)

   David Ruskin: mild pain   moderate pain   severe pain

   Ira Bradley: mild pain   moderate pain   severe pain

6. Only one of the patients was medicated for pain on Tuesday morning. Which patient was medicated for pain? Should both have received pain medication? Why or why not? Can you think of reasons one of the patients did not receive pain medications?

7. Analgesic medications are grouped as Step 1, Step 2 and Step 3 on the analgesic ladder. To what do these levels refer?

Step	Type of Pain	Type of Analgesics Used
1		
2		
3		

8. Consider the pain medications ordered for each patient. Were the medications consistent with the type of pain the patient was experiencing? What recommendations might you make regarding analgesia for these patients?

9. What additional nonpharmacologic pain relief strategies would be appropriate for you, as a student nurse, to offer to Ira Bradley and David Ruskin?

Patient	Nonpharmacologic Strategies
David Ruskin	
Ira Bradley	

10. Before you walk into David Ruskin's room, you hear him laughing. When you enter, you see that he has visitors from the university. When you ask him to rate his pain, he tells you his pain is 8/10. What should you record?
    a. "Pain rating 8/10."
    b. "Pain rating 7/10."
    c. "Pain rating 6/10."
    d. "Patient states 8/10, but this is probably not accurate rating."

11. Oxycodone hydrochloride 5 to 10 mg PO (immediate release) has been ordered for David Ruskin for moderate pain. If you give him a 5-mg dose, what approximate equivalent does this represent?
    a. Morphine 10 mg PO
    b. Morphine 5 mg IM
    c. Codeine 30 mg PO
    d. Codeine 60 mg PO

12. If you administer to David Ruskin oxycodone hydrochloride 5 to 10 mg PO (immediate release) at 0800, approximately what time would it reach peak effect?
    a. 0815
    b. 0830
    c. 0900
    d. 1000

13. Ira Bradley has a pain rating of 9/10. What medication should be offered to him?
    a. Morphine 2 to 8 mg IV
    b. Morphine 30 mg PO
    c. Tylenol 600 mg PO
    d. Oxycodone 10 mg PO

14. Ira Bradley is not sure he wants pain medication because he is concerned about addiction. Which of the following responses by the nurse would be best in this situation?
    a. "I am glad you are concerned about this. Let me know when you really need the medication."
    b. "Since your condition is terminal, addiction is the last thing you should be concerned about."
    c. "Although you may become addicted, we have medications available to help you overcome the addiction."
    d. "Addiction is a common concern patients have, but the truth is, less than 0.1% of people who take pain medication for medical therapy become addicted."

LESSON **9** ——————————————————————————

Inflammation and Infection

———————————————————————————————————

 Reading Assignment: Nursing Management: Inflammation and Infection (Chapter 11)
Patient: Carmen Gonzales, Room 302

Carmen Gonzales was admitted to the hospital on Sunday with a gangrene infection and osteomyelitis to the lower left leg. In the following activities, you will apply the concepts of infection and inflammation as you consider nursing care for this patient.

 Writing Activity

1. Before you begin, answer the following general question: How does a bacterial infection cause lethal cell injury?

CD-ROM Activity

Go to the Supervisor's Office and sign in to work with Carmen Gonzales on Tuesday at 0700. Proceed to the Nurses' Station and open the patient's chart. Read the Physical & History section, including the Emergency Room Record, and answer the following questions.

2. Besides gangrene and osteomyelitis, what other three medical diagnoses are identified upon admission?

   a.

   b.

   c.

3. What are Carmen Gonzales' symptoms upon presentation to the Emergency Department?

4. What are her vital signs at admission?

   Temperature _____ Heart rate _____ Respiratory rate _____ Blood pressure _____

5. What is the relationship between the leg infection and the clinical findings? How can these findings be explained? Below and on the next page, explain the cause and meaning of each of the findings listed.

Clinical Findings	Cause and Meaning of Findings
Fever	
Increased heart rate and respiratory rate	
Malaise, nausea, and anorexia	

Clinical Findings	**Cause and Meaning of Findings**

Pain in the leg

6. In the Emergency Department Record, the physician describes an area of necrosis on the medial side of her left leg. What does the term *necrosis* mean?

 7. What is a common cause of gangrenous necrosis? (Refer to Table 11-4 in your textbook.) Is there any correlation between Carmen Gonzales' other medical problems and the development of gangrenous necrosis? If so, what might that correlation be?

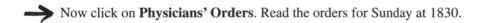 Now click on **Physicians' Orders**. Read the orders for Sunday at 1830.

8. The physician ordered a complete blood count (CBC) and a wound culture on Sunday at 1830. What is the rationale for these tests?

9. Note this order on Sunday evening: "Op permit for surgical debridement . . . ." What is a surgical debridement? Why is the physician going to do this?

10. Find a physician order for wound care in post-op orders on Monday. Record that wound care order below.

11. What is your opinion regarding the dressing change order? What additional information would you expect? What seems to be missing?

12. Close the chart. Go to the computer under the bookshelf and open the EPR for Carmen Gonzales. Click on **Hematology** and record the CBC and differential results for Sunday evening below.

Lab Test	Result	Lab Test	Result
Hgb		Neutrophil segs %	
Hct		Neutrophil bands %	
RBC		Lymphocytes %	
Platelets		Monocytes %	
WBC		Eosinophils %	
		Dasophils %	

 Which of the results are abnormal? Circle each abnormal result and indicate whether it is high or low. What is your interpretation of the CBC results? Do any of these results surprise you? (Refer to Appendix B in your textbook for help.)

→ Close the EPR. Now go to the blue notebook on the counter and open the MAR for Carmen Gonzales.

13. What medication is being given on Tuesday for Carmen Gonzales' infection? Fill in the missing data in the medication order below.

_____   _____ grams   IVPG   q _____ hours
    (name of medication)   (dose)   (route)   (frequency)

Times the medication is due on Tuesday: _____ _____ _____ _____

14. What other two medications can the nurse administer to help treat symptoms associated with the inflammatory process? When should they be given?

Medication and Dose	Given for What Reason? How often?
Acetaminophen 650 mg PO	
Morphine 2 to 5 mg IM	
Oxycodone 10 mg PO	

15. Before you administer a medication, you must be familiar with that agent. Fill out the following drug card for cefoxitin. (You will probably need to refer to your nursing drug book.)

Cefoxitin Drug Card

Classification:

Action:

Indications:

Contraindications/Precautions:

Major Adverse Effects:

Typical Dose:

IV Administration:

---

16. Close the MAR. Consider the nursing interventions discussed in the textbook. Nursing interventions include fever management, administration of antibiotics to treat the infection, wound management, and pain management. What other nursing measures should be included in your plan of care for Carmen Gonzales? Provide a rationale for each of your planned measures.

Nursing Measure	Rationale

17. Refer to Carmen Gonzales' CBC differential count results you recorded earlier in this lesson. Which of the following explains why the eosinophils are not elevated?
    a. Eosinophils are chronically low in patients with diabetes.
    b. An increase in eosinophils is usually associated with allergic reaction.
    c. Eosinophils are never elevated in the presence of anemia.
    d. An increase in neutrophils causes phagocytosis of eosinophils.

18. Carmen Gonzales had purulent drainage from her wound infection. Which of the following describes the cause of exudate formation?
    a. Cellular lysis from bacterial invasion and destruction
    b. Fluid and leukocytes move to the site of infection
    c. Cellular release of histamine
    d. Fluid shift from intracellular to extracelluar space

19. It is 0700 on Tuesday morning. Carmen Gonzales' vital signs are as follows: Temp 102.6° F, HR 108, RR 22, and BP 138/88. Which of the following nursing measures is most appropriate in response to this data?
    a. Elevate the patient's left leg.
    b. Change the dressing on the wound.
    c. Administer the antibiotic cefoxitin now.
    d. Administer acetaminophen now.

20. The nurse anticipates that Carmen Gonzales may experience delayed wound healing for which of the following reasons?
    a. She has diabetes.
    b. She had a surgical debridement.
    c. She had a lot of pain in the leg.
    d. She had an elevated WBC.

21. In order to reduce the spread of infection to this patient, which of the following nursing measures, in addition to handwashing, should be followed?
    a. Wear eye protection and a mask (or face shield) during dressing changes.
    b. Use sterile linens when making the patient's bed.
    c. Follow meticulous aseptic technique during dressing changes to her leg.
    d. Place the patient in protective isolation.

10 ——————————————————————

HIV—Part I

———————————————————————————————————

 Reading Assignment: Nursing Management: Human Immunodeficiency Virus Infection
(Chapter 13)
Patient: Ira Bradley, Room 309

You have been assigned to care for Ira Bradley, a 41-year-old man admitted to the hospital on Sunday with late-stage HIV, *Pneumocystis carinii* pneumonia, candidiasis, and Kaposi's sarcoma. In order to provide competent care, you must first prepare by reading his chart and considering care as outlined in your textbook.

 CD-ROM Activity

Go to the Supervisor's Office and sign in to work with Ira Bradley for the Tuesday 0700 shift. Proceed to the Nurses' Station and open the patient's chart. Read the Physical & History, including the Emergency Department Report. Click on **Physicians' Orders** and read the orders for Sunday. Answer the following questions, based on what you have read.

Writing Activity

1. Ira Bradley has had an HIV infection for several years. What was the primary reason his wife brought him to the hospital on Sunday?

2. Based on data in the chart, circle the HIV infection phase below that is consistent with Ira Bradley's condition. Provide a rationale based on criteria found in your textbook.

HIV Infection Phase	Rationale
Acute retroviral syndrome	
Early infection (asymptomatic)	
Early symptomatic disease	
AIDS	

3. According to the Emergency Department Report, the physician suspected several opportunistic infections and diseases. For each of these conditions, compare Ira Bradley's situation (according to the ER records and initial admission orders) with textbook descriptions in the following three areas: clinical findings, diagnostic tests, and treatment initiated. (Refer to Table 13-2 in the textbook for help.)

Opportunistic Disease/Infection	Clinical Findings	
	Typical Findings According to Textbook	Ira Bradley's Findings
Pneumocystis carinii pneumonia		
Kaposi's sarcoma		
Candida (oral candidiasis)		

Opportunistic Disease/Infection	Diagnostic Tests	
	Typical Tests According to Textbook	**Ira Bradley's Tests**
Pneumocystis carinii pneumonia		
Kaposi's sarcoma		
Candida (oral candidiasis)		

Opportunistic Disease/Infection	Treatment (Medications)	
	Typical Treatment According to Textbook	**Ira Bradley's Treatment**
Pneumocystis carinii pneumonia		
Kaposi's sarcoma		
Candida (oral candidiasis)		

4. Consider the figure below showing a timeline spectrum of HIV infection. How does Ira Bradley's condition compare with this figure based on what you know?

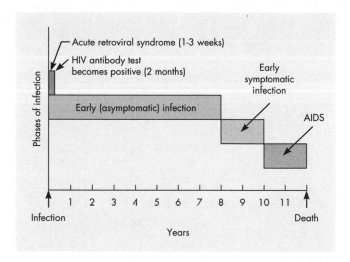

Now click on **Nurses' Notes** in Ira Bradley's chart. Read the notes for Sunday, Monday, and Tuesday morning.

5. What pattern of change is noted over the last few shifts?

→ Close the chart. Click on the computer below the bookshelf and open Ira Bradley's EPR.

6. Review the vital signs taken since admission. What sorts of patterns do you see in Ira Bradley's vital signs over the course of the last couple of days?

7. Review the pain assessment since admission. What sorts of patterns do you see in Ira Bradley's level and type of pain over the course of the last couple of days?

8. Check Ira Bradley's CBC and chemistry lab results from Sunday night. Record the results below and on the next page. Circle any abnormal findings and indicate whether the result is higher or lower than normal range. In the right-hand column, indicate the significance of any of these findings. The first one is done for you.

Lab Test	Result	What does it reflect?
Sodium	(152) (high)	Hypernatremia consistent with dehydration
Potassium		
Chloride		
CO_2		
BUN		
Creatinine		
Albumin		
Hemoglobin		

Lab Test	Result	What does it reflect?
Hematocrit		
RBCs		
Platelets		

➡ Close the EPR. Now go to the MAR and open Ira Bradley's record. Review the routine medications he is receiving.

9. Using your textbook and a drug reference, determine the classification of each drug ordered for Ira Bradley (listed below and on the next page) and provide a reason that the drug has been ordered. Check to verify that the dosage and route are within recommended guidelines.

Medication, Dose, Route	Classification	Reason Ordered
D₅ 0.45 NS @ 125 cc/hour	*Intravenous fluid Hypotonic*	*Pt. dehydrated upon admission – would use this solution to rehydrate would h*
AZT 1 mg/kg IVPB over 1h, q4h x 24 doses	*Antiviral agent*	*Used in combo c̄ other anti-retroviral agents in TX of HIV infection*
Trimethoprim 300 mg and sulfamethoxazole 1.5 g IVPB q6h x 16 doses	*Antibacterial antiprotozoal*	*Used to treat Pneumocystis carinii pneumonitis*

Medication, Dose, Route	Classification	Reason Ordered
Delavirdine myselate 400 mg PO TID *Dose ok*	*antiretroviral agent*	*used in conjunction ō other antiviral in TX of HIV inf.*
Saquinovir 1200 mg PO TID within 2h of eating *OK dose*	*antiretroviral agent*	*used in conj. with other antiviral in tx HIV inf.*
Fluconazole 100 mg PO in A.M. x 14 days *OK dose*	*antifungal*	*used to treat candidiasis*
Alitretinoin gel 0.1%, apply to lesions, BID *OK Dose*	*antisporeatus*	*TX of lesions from AIDS-related Kaposi sarcoma*
Hydroxyurea	*ō antineoplastic*	*used as part of antiretroviral therapy in pt ō HIV inf.*

10. Why are three antiretroviral agents included in the routine medications given to Ira Bradley? What is the advantage of administering three as opposed to just one?

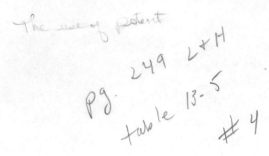

11. Consider Ira Bradley's condition and physician orders. What type of precautions must the nurse take to prevent spread of HIV to himself or herself, as well as to other patients? What infection control concerns should the nurse have on behalf of Ira Bradley?

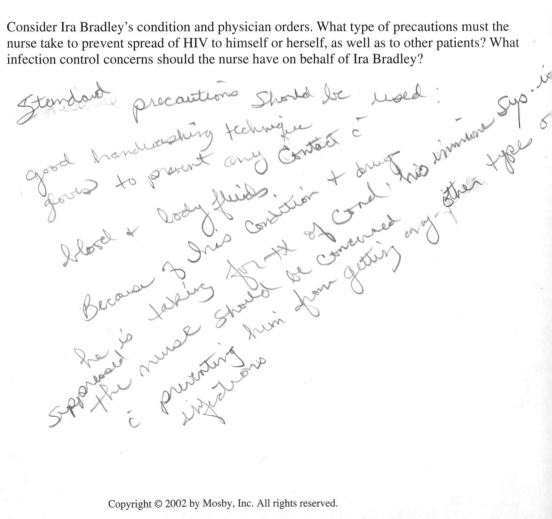

12. When Ira Bradley arrived to the Emergency Department on Sunday, the nurse recorded the following vital signs: Temp 100.1° F, BP 105/75, RR 23, HR 95, O_2 sat 85% on room air. Based on these findings, which of the following interventions should the nurse take immediately?
    a. Administer acetaminophen for the fever.
    b. Place Ira Bradley in the supine position with his legs elevated.
    c. Start an IV line.
    d. Administer oxygen.

13. Which of the following laboratory tests is frequently used to evaluate the status and guide treatment of a patient with HIV infection but has not been ordered for Ira Bradley?
    a. CD4+ T cell count
    b. Blood cultures
    c. Lung tissue biopsy
    d. Stool culture

14. Ira Bradley was in the hospital 6 weeks ago for *Pneumocystis carinii* pneumonia. This fact supports which of the following statements?
    a. He has not been compliant with his medication regime.
    b. The infection from 6 weeks ago has now spread to his mouth.
    c. The HIV agents he is taking are not effective.
    d. These infections tend to be cyclical because they usually are not fully eradicated.

15. The initial disorientation Ira Bradley experienced during the first few days of hospitalization can best be explained by:
    a. cryptococcal meningitis.
    b. closed head injury from the fall.
    c. fluid and electrolyte imbalances.
    d. side effects of antiretroviral therapy.

16. At this point in time, which of the following focuses of care seem to be most applicable?
    a. Patient and family teaching regarding prevention of HIV transmission (e.g., using sterile linens when making the patient's bed)
    b. Identification of social and financial support for the patient and family
    c. Discussion with patient and family regarding progress in the development of the HIV vaccine
    d. Discussion with the family regarding the possible use of restraints

HIV—Part II

_____

 Reading Assignment: Nursing Management: Human Immunodeficiency Virus Infection
(Chapter 13)
Patient: Ira Bradley, Room 309

In this lesson, you will continue to care for Ira Bradley, a 41-year-old man admitted to the hospital on Sunday with late-stage HIV, *Pneumocystis carinii* pneumonia, candidiasis, and Kaposi's sarcoma. In Lesson 10, you prepared by reading his chart and considering his care as outlined in your textbook. In this lesson, you will participate in the patient's care.

 CD-ROM Activity

Go to the Supervisor's Office and sign in to work with Ira Bradley for the Tuesday 0700 shift. Proceed to the Nurses' Station and check the bulletin board to determine where report is being given for this patient. Go to that location and listen to the report.

Writing Activity

1. As you listen to the report on Ira Bradley, record pertinent information using the form on the following page.

Red Rock Canyon Medical Center
Report Notes

Patient: _____ Room # _____

Age: _____ Diagnosis: _____

Vital signs: _____ O$_2$ sat:_____ Pain: _____

Treatments:

Significant assessment findings:

IV location/date: _____

Identified patient/family problems:

2. What did you think of the report? What information was not given by the nurse that you think should have been included? What information were you given that you did not find helpful?

3. It is now 0730. Go to the MAR in the Nurses' Station. Click open Ira Bradley's MAR and identify the medications you will need to give him this morning. For each of the medications listed below, record the times that drug is due today between 0800 and 1500.

Routine medications, dose, and route	Time due	PRN medications given since midnight last night (including dose and time given)
AZT 1 mg/kg IVPB over 1 hour, q4h x 24 doses		
Trimethoprim 300 mg and sulfamethoxazole 1.5 g IVPB q6h x 16 doses		
Delavirdine myselate 400 mg PO TID		
Saquinovir 1200 mg PO TID within 2 hours of eating		
Fluconazole 100 mg PO A.M. x 14 days		
Alitretinoin gel 0.1%, apply to lesions BID		

4. It is now 0800. The primary nurse tells you she will take care of the 0800 medications while you obtain a set of vital signs. Go into Ira Bradley's room and click on **Vital Signs**. Obtain a full set of vital signs and record them below.

Blood pressure _____   Heart rate _____

Respiration _____   Temperature _____

Oxygen saturation _____   Pain location _____

Pain characteristics _____   Level of pain   1 2 3 4 5 6 7 8 9 10

5. Is Ira Bradley wearing oxygen at the time the oxygen saturation is taken?

6. Is the use of oxygen significant when documenting oxygen saturation levels? Why or why not? What should be recorded when documenting oxygen saturation?

7. Based on the vital signs, write the appropriate three-part nursing diagnosis evident at this time and some appropriate nursing interventions.

Nursing Diagnosis	**Interventions**
_____	
related to _____	
_____	
_____	
as manifested by _____	
_____	
_____	

8. It is now 0830—time to conduct your bedside nursing assessment. Click on **Physical Assessment** and obtain data from the physical examination. Record your findings below and on the next page. Circle any findings that are considered abnormal.

Examination	**Findings**
Head and Neck	

Examination   **Findings**

Chest/
Upper Extremities

Abdomen and
Lower Extremities

9. Based on the data you heard in report earlier this morning, there are a couple of other things
   the nurse should have included during the examination—one involving the upper extremities and one involving the lower extremities. What is missing?

   Upper extremities

   Lower extremities

→ It is 0900—time to give medications. While in Ira Bradley's room, click on **Medications**. Now click on **Review Medications**, and a pop-up box will appear, listing medications the nurse is preparing to administer. Next, click on **Administer**, and you will see the nurse giving him his medications.

10. a. Which medication is the nursing giving 1 hour later than indicated on the MAR?

b. Is this a serious issue? Why or why not?

c. How should this be documented on the MAR?

d. What further action by the nurse is appropriate?

11. a. What medication is due at 0900 but does not appear on the pop-up box while the nurse is administering medications?

   b. Where is a medication like this frequently kept?

   c. What is a likely explanation for not seeing this medication given at this time?

➡ 12. It is now 1000. While still in Ira Bradley's room, click on **Health History**. Record significant data below and on the next two pages.

Area	Data
Perception/ Self-Concept	
Activity	

Area	Data
Sexuality/Reproduction	
Culture	
Nutrition/Metabolic	
Sleep/Rest	

Area	Data
Role/Relationship	
Health Perception	
Elimination	
Cognitive/Perceptual	

Area	Data
Coping/Stress	
Values/Beliefs	

 13. Review ongoing care in the Ambulatory and Home Care section in your textbook. How are the concepts presented in these sections relevant to Ira Bradley?

14. Based on your interview, examination findings, and information from the chart, develop a list of nursing diagnoses and collaborative problems for Ira Bradley. Be sure you can support all of the problems you select with data. Use your textbook for additional help.

Nursing Diagnoses	**Collaborative Problems**

15. From the problem list you developed in question 14, choose two problems and develop them further. For each problem, identify patient outcomes and nursing interventions specific for Ira Bradley. Why did you select the ones that you did?

Nursing Diagnosis or Collaborative Problem	Outcomes	Nursing Interventions

LESSON 12

Cancer

 Reading Assignment: Nursing Management: Cancer (Chapter 14)
Patient: Ira Bradley, Room 309

Once again, you have been assigned to care for Ira Bradley. Remember that he is a 41-year-old man admitted to the hospital on Sunday with late-stage HIV, *Pneumocystis carinii* pneumonia, candidiasis, and Kaposi's sarcoma.

Before you begin working with Ira Bradley, review a few concepts associated with cancer.

Writing Activity

1. Briefly describe what is meant by the following three stages in the development of cancer.

Cancer Stage	Description
Initiation	The 1st Stage in Ca. pg 272
Promotion	274

Cancer Stage	Description
Progression	

2. The textbook describes the immune system role in the recognition and destruction of tumor cells. Briefly describe the response to tumor-associated antigens (TAAs) by immunologic surveillance.

Malignant causes A on Cancer Cell surface antigen. Called Tumor associated antigens (TAA's). During immunol. Sur. lymphocytes constantly check the cell surface antigens and find + destroy any unusual. Usually any one who has a normal functioning immune response this surveillance mechanism will keep cancer cells from becoming detectable tumors.

3. Briefly describe the following four specific immune responses to tumor cells.

Immune Response	Description
Cytotoxic T cells	*act in combatting tumor growth. Also important because they produce cytokines such as interleukin 2 and γ-interferon. These cytokines, in turn cause the stimulation of T cells, nat kill cells + macrophages, which are also important cells of the immune response.*
Natural killer cells (NK)	*These are cells that are stimulated by the Cytotoxic T cells. Can automatically destroy tumor cells ŝ having to be stimulated beforehand.*

Immune Response	Description
Macrophages	

277

B-lymphocytes

4. One of Ira Bradley's admitting diagnoses is Kaposi's sarcoma (KS) on the left leg. What is KS?

pg 504

5. According to the textbook, the types of cancer found in immunosuppressed individuals are primarily epithelial or lymphoid. Is this statement consistent with Ira Bradley's condition? If so, in what way?

CD-ROM Activity

Go to the Supervisor's Office and sign in to work with Ira Bradley for the Tuesday 0700 shift. Your first task is to collect data. Specifically, you are interested in data associated with KS. Proceed to the Nurses' Station and open Ira Bradley's EPR. Read his Admissions Profile, taking notes as you read.

6. What information is found in the profile related to KS?

Notes from Admissions Profile

Close the EPR and open Ira Bradley's chart. Read the Physical & History, including the Emergency Department Report.

7. What mention is made of KS in the Physical & History? Is there any indication of current or recent past treatment for this condition?

Notes from Physical & History

 Now click on **Physicians' Orders**.

 8. What orders are directly related to the treatment of KS? How does this compare with the typical medical intervention? In the left-hand column below, indicate the current orders, if any, for treatment of KS in Ira Bradley's chart. In the right-hand column, describe the typical treatment for KS affecting the integumentary system (according to your textbook).

Orders for Ira Bradley   **Treatment According to Textbook**

9. According to the textbook, there are three primary goals of cancer care. Circle the goal of care that is most appropriate for Ira Bradley at this point. Provide a rationale for your answer.

Cure   Control   Palliation

10. Refer to the Patient with Cancer care plan in your textbook. Indicate which of the following nursing diagnoses are applicable to Ira Bradley's situation. For those not applicable as written, suggest modifications to make them specific to his needs.

Nursing Diagnosis	Applicable as Is? (Yes or No)	Suggested Modification
Altered oral mucous membrane related to chemotherapy or radiation		
Fatigue related to effects of cancer		

Nursing Diagnosis	Applicable as Is? (Yes or No)	Suggested Modification
Ineffective individual coping related to depression secondary to diagnosis and treatment		
Body-image disturbance related to hair loss, disfiguring surgery and weight loss		
Altered family processes related to cancer diagnosis of family member		

Fluid and Electrolyte Imbalance—Part I: Preclinical Preparation

 Reading Assignment: Nursing Management: Fluid, Electrolyte, and Acid-Base
Imbalances (Chapter 15)

Patient: Ira Bradley, Room 309

In this lesson, you will continue to care for Ira Bradley. Now you are interested in learning about his fluid and electrolyte status upon admission and the initial treatment for this.

 CD-ROM Activity

Go to the Supervisor's Office and sign in to work with Ira Bradley for the Tuesday 0700 shift. Proceed to the Nurses' Station and open his chart. Read the entire Physical & History, including the Emergency Department Report.

Writing Activity

1. Below and on the next page, list data you found in the Emergency Department Report and other sections of the Physical & History that suggest a possible fluid and electrolyte imbalance. Are the findings consistent?

Emergency Department Report

Physical & History

2. The physician indicates Ira Bradley is dehydrated. What events most likely led to this condition?

➡ Now click on **Nurses' Notes** and read the note documented by T. Landers at 2335 Sunday.

3. What subjective and objective data are found, if any, that address Ira Bradley's fluid and electrolyte status?

Subjective Data

Objective Data

➡ Next, click on **Physicians' Orders** and read the orders for Sunday at 2255.

4. What lab tests were ordered that could provide important information regarding fluid and electrolyte status? In the presence of dehydration, what results are expected?

Lab tests useful for assessing fluid and electrolyte status	Expected results in presence of dehydration

5. In addition to the lab tests, what other orders written on Sunday night are specific interventions to manage dehydration?

➡ Close the chart and open Ira Bradley's EPR.

6. Find the lab results for the CBC, albumin, Chem 7, and urinalysis that were done on Sunday evening. Record the findings in the table below. Then indicate whether each value is low (L), high (H), or in the normal range (N). Finally, indicate what you think might be causing the change in value, if applicable.

Lab	Value	L, H, N	Meaning
Na$^+$			
K$^+$			
Cl$^-$			
CO$_2$			
BUN			
Creatinine			
Albumin			

Lab	Value	L, H, N	Meaning
Hgb			
Hct			
Urine specific gravity			

 7. Look at the figure below from your textbook. Based on the information you have collected so far, circle the box that best represents the pathology of Ira Bradley's fluid and electrolyte condition upon admission. Then circle the appropriate description of the cause of the problem.

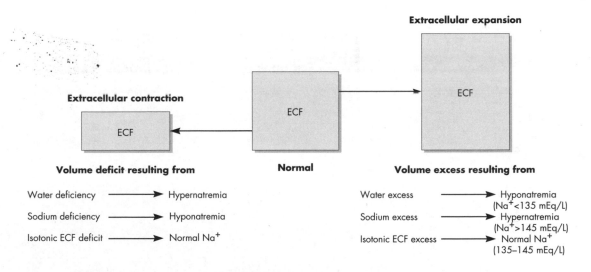

8. Ira Bradley has experienced a fluid shift. Fill in the sodium level in the space below. Next, draw an arrow indicating the direction of fluid shift between the extracellular space and the intracellular space.

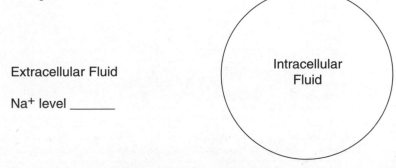

Extracellular Fluid

Na+ level _____

Intracellular Fluid

Refer to your textbook regarding collaborative care in the treatment of hypernatremia to answer the following questions.

9. What is the primary goal of treatment?

10. Compare the treatment described in the textbook with Ira Bradley's orders.

Treatment	Textbook	Ira Bradley's Orders
Route of fluid replacement		
Type of IV fluid		

Now, consider intake and output (I&O).

11. What would you anticipate the I&O records to reflect over the first 24 to 48 hours of hospitalization? What would be a reasonable guess as to the intake verses the output? Would you expect these to be nearly equal?

12. What did the I&O actually look like? With the EPR still open, click on **I&O**. Record intake and output totals for the following time frames:

	Sunday Admission to 2400	Sunday 2400 to Monday 0800	Monday 0800 to 1600	Totals
Intake Totals				
Output Totals				

13. Are the totals similar to what you expected? How do the above totals compare with what you expected? How can you explain these totals?

→ Now click on **Assessment** (still in the EPR). Review the assessments completed by the nursing staff from admission until now (Tuesday 0700).

14. What data can be found that addresses the fluid and electrolyte status? From this standpoint, do you think the documentation is adequate? What could have been and/or should have been included as part of the nursing assessment?

→ Close the EPR. Go back to Ira Bradley's chart and review physicians' notes, physicians' orders, and nurses' notes from Sunday night until now, Tuesday morning.

15. What documentation and changes in orders, if any, reflect a change in the patient's care concerning his dehydration? Do any of the data seem surprising to you? If so, which? Record your answers below and on the next page.

Physicians' Notes   Monday:

Tuesday:

Physicians' Orders   Monday:

Tuesday:

Nurses' Notes   Monday:

Tuesday:

Fluid and Electrolyte Imbalance—Part II

📖 **Reading Assignment:** Nursing Management: Fluid, Electrolyte, and Acid-Base Imbalances (Chapter 15)

Patient: Ira Bradley, Room 309

In Lesson 13 you completed preclinical preparation for Ira Bradley, a 41-year-old man admitted to the hospital on Sunday with late-stage HIV infection, *Pneumocystis carinii* pneumonia, candidiasis, and Kaposi's sarcoma (KS). That lesson focused on the patient's fluid and electrolyte status upon admission and his initial treatment. In this lesson you will continue to follow this case as Ira Bradley recovers from dehydration.

💿 **CD-ROM Activity**

Go to the Supervisor's Office and sign in to work with Ira Bradley for the Tuesday 0700 shift. Proceed to the Nurses' Station and check the bulletin board to determine where report is being given for this patient. Go to that location and listen to the nursing report.

1. Below, record pertinent information from report regarding fluid and electrolyte status.

➡ Return to the Nurses' Station and open the MAR (in the blue notebook on the countertop).

2. What is the IV fluid and infusion rate being administered at this time?

3. What is the physiologic effect of this IV fluid?

4. If you have a 20 gtt/cc administration set, what is the correct drip rate (gtts/minute) to deliver the IV fluid at the ordered infusion rate?

5. If you know that a new liter of IV fluid was hung at 0400 this morning, about what time should you anticipate this liter will be empty?

→ Go to Ira Bradley's room to conduct the physical examination.

6. Record physical examination findings below. Include data that you think provide some information about fluid and electrolyte status. Also explain *how* each finding relates to fluid and electrolyte assessment.

Assessment findings related to fluid and electrolyte status	How do findings relate to fluid and electrolyte assessment?

7. What additional assessment would you perform to gain further information regarding the progress of Ira Bradley's hydration status or related treatment?

8. Your nursing instructor encourages you to consider using the nursing diagnosis Fluid volume deficit for your plan of care. Write this as a three-part nursing diagnosis.

Fluid volume deficit related to:

as manifested by:

9. One of the goals for Ira Bradley is rehydration. Interventions to accomplish this goal include administration of intravenous infusion of fluids and increased oral fluid intake. Considering these efforts, answer the following questions:

   a. What are some nursing interventions that can help increase the oral fluid intake, given the infection in his mouth?

   b. In what way does the management of Ira Bradley's fever, episodic diarrhea, and shortness of breath contribute to rehydration efforts?

   c. In what ways could you evaluate the effectiveness of the rehydration efforts?

→ It is now Friday and you have returned to the hospital to follow up on Ira Bradley. You are specifically interested in his fluid and electrolyte status and how his care may have changed since Tuesday. In the Supervisor's Office, sign in to work with him again, selecting Friday 0700 as your shift. Go to the Nurses' Station and open Ira Bradley's chart. Review the physicians' orders, physicians' notes, and nurses' notes for any indication regarding his condition, change in status, or change in orders that specifically address the fluid and electrolyte imbalance.

10. Record your findings below and on the next page.

Day	Data	Source (physicians' notes, physicians' orders, nurses' notes)
Tuesday		Physicians' notes
		Physicians' orders
		Nurses' notes
Wednesday		Physicians' notes
		Physicians' orders
		Nurses' notes

Day	Data	Source (physicians' notes, physicians' orders, nurses' notes)
Thursday		Physicians' notes
		Physicians' orders
		Nurses' notes

→ Close the patient's chart and move to the computer under the bookshelf. Access Ira Bradley's EPR and review his electrolytes and urine specific gravity over the entire week. (You will need to click on **Chemistry** and **Urinalysis** to find this data.)

11. Record your findings below and explain any changes in the data.

Test	Sunday	Tuesday	Thursday
Na^+			
K^+			
Cl^-			
CO_2			
BUN			
Creatinine			
Urine specific gravity			

Explanation for changes:

12. Now look at the intake and output totals over the entire week. Fill in the 24-hour I&O totals below. Explain any changes in the data.

Day	Intake totals	Output totals
Sunday		
Monday		
Tuesday		
Wednesday		
Thursday		

Explanation of changes:

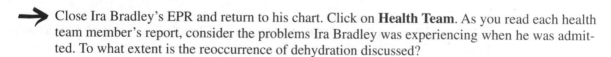 Close Ira Bradley's EPR and return to his chart. Click on **Health Team**. As you read each health team member's report, consider the problems Ira Bradley was experiencing when he was admitted. To what extent is the reoccurrence of dehydration discussed?

13. Below and on the next page, indicate what each of the three health team members reported, if anything, regarding hydration.

Health Team Member	Information in Report Regarding Hydration
Sara Terney	

Health Team Member	Information in Report Regarding Hydration
Ray Burns	
Bridget Natalicio	

14. What strategies can you think of that would reduce Ira Bradley's chances of dehydration in the future?

LESSON **15**

Perioperative Care

✐ **Reading Assignment:** Nursing Management: Preoperative Patient (Chapter 16)
Nursing Management: Patient During Surgery (Chapter 17)
Nursing Management: Postoperative Patient (Chapter 18)
Patient: David Ruskin, Room 303

In this lesson, you will be considering the perioperative experience of David Ruskin, who was struck by a motor vehicle while riding a bicycle, suffering a fractured right humerus and a closed head injury.

💿 **CD-ROM Activity**

Go to the Supervisor's Office and sign in to work with David Ruskin for the Tuesday 0700 shift. Proceed to the Nurses' Station and open his chart. Read the Emergency Department Report in the Physical & History section.

  1. What time did David Ruskin present to the Emergency Department?

  2. What time did he go to surgery?

📖 Review in your textbook the two categories of surgery.

  3. Which type of surgery did David Ruskin have—elective or emergency? *(Circle one.)*

  4. According to the textbook, three conditions must be met to obtain a valid consent for surgery.

    a. What are these three conditions? 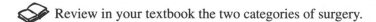 ρ𝓈' 3⁶⁷

b. Why did David Ruskin's wife Lisa sign the operative permit instead of David?

5. Your textbook describes several common fears associated with surgery. Which of the following, if any, are documented fears that David Ruskin had before going into surgery? (Place an **X** next to all that apply.)

_____ Fear of pain

_____ Fear of the unknown

_____ Fear of death

_____ Fear of anesthesia

_____ Fear of disruption of life patterns

 6. Read the section on assessment of the preoperative patient in your textbook. How does this compare with David Ruskin's preoperative assessment? Why are there differences?

7. If you had been the ER nurse caring for David Ruskin, what preoperative teaching would you have provided? How would his level of consciousness have affected your teaching?

 8. Many patients receive preoperative medications, sometimes a single drug, sometimes a combination of drugs. Listed below and on the next page are common types of preoperative medications discussed in your textbook. Indicate the purpose for which these drugs are given.

Medication	Purpose
Benzodiazepines and barbiturates	
Anticholinergics	
Narcotics	

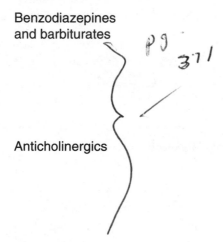

Medication	Purpose
Antiemetics	
Antibiotics	
Low-dose heparin	

3 71

➡ Review the physicians' orders in David Ruskin's chart.

9. Which of the medications listed in question 8 were administered to this patient before his surgery?

➡ Now review the surgeons' notes for David Ruskin.

10. According to the surgeons' notes, what time was he brought into the operating room?

11. What time did his surgery actually begin?

12. What surgical procedure was performed on David Ruskin?

13. How was the patient's fracture repaired?

14. What time did the surgical procedure end?

 According to the report, David Ruskin was transferred to the Postanesthesia Care Unit (PACU) at 1855. Refer to your textbook to answer the following questions.

 15. When a patient is admitted to the PACU, the major initial priority is assessment. What specific priorities are associated with this assessment?

39°

16. In the PACU, nurses monitor for common respiratory complications such as airway obstruction, hypoxemia, and hypoventilation. What is the most common source of airway obstruction immediately after general anesthesia? What is the most common cause of hypoxemia?

392

393

17. What criteria must be met before a patient can be discharged from the PACU and transferred to the nursing unit?

Table 18-4
pg 399

→ David Ruskin was transferred from the PACU to the nursing unit at 2000. Immediately upon receiving this patient, the nurse performed an assessment. In David Ruskin's chart, read the nurses' notes for Sunday at 2030. Then close the chart and open David Ruskin's EPR. Click on **Assessment** and read the documentation regarding his initial postoperative assessment.

18. Compare the data you read in the nurses' notes and EPR with that shown in the table below from your textbook. What is your opinion of the assessment data documented by the nurses on the unit? Are their findings consistent with what is suggested in the table? Place a check mark next to each item below that is documented either in the EPR or the nurses' notes.

Table 15-1   Nursing Assessment and Care of Patient on Admission to Clinical Unit

- Record time of patient's return to unit
- Take baseline vital signs
    Assess airway and breath sounds
- Assess neurologic status, including level of consciousness and movement of extremities
- Assess wound, dressing, drainage tubes
    Note type and amount of drainage
    Connect tubing to gravity or suction drainage
- Assess color and appearance of skin
- Assess urinary status
    Note time of voiding
    Note presence of catheter and total output
    Check for bladder distention or urge to void
    Note catheter patency
- Assess pain and discomfort
    Note last dose and type of pain control
    Note current pain intensity
- Position for airway maintenance, comfort, safety (bed in low position, side rails up)
- Check IV infusion
    Note type of solution
    Note amount of fluid remaining
    Note flow rate
    Check integrity of insertion site and size of catheter
- Attach call light within reach and reorient patient to use of call light
- Ensure that emesis basin and tissues are available
- Determine emotional condition and support
    Check for presence of family member or significant other
- Check and carry out postoperative orders

→ After completing an assessment, the nurse caring for David Ruskin should immediately review the physicians' orders and initiate a plan of care. Go back to the patient's chart, click on **Physicians' Orders** and read the Sunday 1930 postoperative orders. Next, review the Postoperative Care Plan in your textbook.

19. Based on the nursing postoperative assessment and physicians' orders, which of the following nursing diagnoses and collaborative problems seem applicable in David Ruskin's situation? (Circle all that apply.)

Nursing Diagnoses	Collaborative Problems
Pain	PC: Thromboembolism
Risk for infection	PC: Paralytic ileu
Anxiety	PC: Hemorrhage
Nausea	PC: Urinary retention
Ineffective airway clearance	
Risk for constipation	

pg 401

20. What additional problems (nursing diagnoses or collaborative problems) would you include?

pg 1780 Ft Nursing Care Plan
pg 1628 Head inj. Diagnoses

LESSON **16**

Pneumonia—Part I: Preclinical Preparation

/⊙⊙ **Reading Assignment:** Nursing Assessment: Respiratory System (Chapter 24)
Nursing Management: Lower Respiratory System (Chapter 26)
Patient: Sally Begay, Room 304

In this lesson, you will complete preclinical preparation for Sally Begay, a 58-year-old Navajo woman with a diagnosis of pneumonia.

🖸 CD-ROM Activity

Go to the Supervisor's Office and sign in to work with Sally Begay for the Tuesday 0700 shift. Proceed to the Nurses' Station and open her chart. In the Physical & History, read the admitting report completed in the Emergency Department at 1200.

1. What was Sally Begay's initial admitting diagnosis?

2. Now scroll down to read the History of Present Illness section of the Physical & History. What are Sally Begay's primary symptoms, and how long has she had these symptoms?

161

3. What other health problems does Sally Begay have, according to her history? (*Hint: Five problems are listed under Significant Medical History.*)

→ An initial possible diagnosis for Sally Begay was Hantavirus. To answer the following questions, you will need to use sources other than your textbook. One good source is the CDC Website on Hantavirus. *(http://www.cdc.gov/ncidod/diseases/hanta/hps/noframes/othrsrce.htm).* You can access this site on the Intranet computer in the Nurses' Station.

4. What is Hantavirus?

5. What data are found in the History of Present Illness section that make the physician suspect the possibility of this diagnosis?

6. Sally Begay is ultimately diagnosed with pneumonia. Your textbook describes two classifications of pneumonia, based on how the infection was acquired. Which type of pneumonia does Sally Begay have?

7. Sally Begay is found to have bacterial pneumonia. Briefly describe the four stages of bacterial pneumonia, as described in your textbook.

Stage	Description
Congestion	
Red hepatization	
Gray hepatization	
Resolution	

8. On the flow sheet below, indicate where each of the four stages (congestion, red hepatization, gray hepatization, and resolution) occur. *(Note: Refer to Figure 26-1 in your textbook if you need help.)*

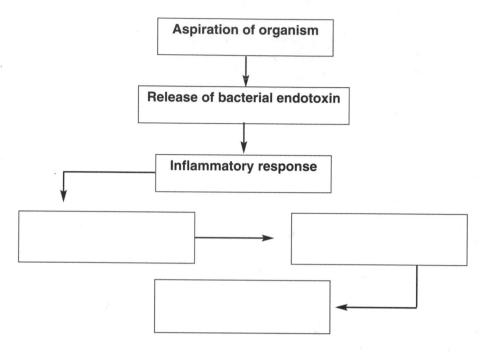

9. Which medical problem found in Sally Begay's medical history is most likely to have contributed to the development of pneumonia?
   a. MI 5 years ago
   b. Angina
   c. Hypertension
   d. Congestive heart failure
   e. COPD—chronic bronchitis

→ Click on **Physicians' Orders** in the patient's chart. Look over the initial orders written at 1230 on Saturday. Compare the diagnostic tests ordered with the common diagnostic measures for pneumonia presented in Table 26-5 in your textbook.

10. Which of the following diagnostic measures were ordered for Sally Begay? (Place an **X** next to all correct answers.)

_____ History and physical examination   _____ ABG

_____ Chest x-ray   _____ CBC

_____ Gram's stain of sputum   _____ Blood cultures

_____ Sputum culture

→ Now click on **Diagnostics** in the chart. Read the CXR report by Dr. Kawasaki.

11. What findings appear on the x-ray that suggest pneumonia?

→ Close the chart and open Sally Begay's EPR (on the computer under the bookshelf).

12. Find the results of the CBC done on Saturday. In the chart below, write the normal value for each test. *(Note: Refer to Appendix B in your textbook for normal lab values.)* Then record Sally Begay's results for each test. Circle any abnormal values.

Test	Normal Value	Sally Begay's Results
Hgb		
Hct		
WBC		
RBC		
Platelets		

13. Now find the results of the ABG done on Saturday. Record Sally Begay's results below, as well as the normal value for each test. *(See Appendix B in your textbook.)* Circle any abnormal values.

Test	Normal Value	Sally Begay's Results
pH		
$PaCO_2$		
PaO_2		
HCO_3		

14. What is the significance of the CBC and ABG results? What do these results reflect?

→ Close the EPR and access Sally Begay's MAR (in the blue notebook on the counter).

15. Listed below are the medications (routine or PRN) ordered specifically to treat Sally Begay's pneumonia. Indicate the classification of each medication and the role you believe it plays in the treatment of pneumonia.

Medication	Type/Classification	Role in Treatment of Pneumonia
Erythromycin		
Ceftizoxime		
Acetaminophen		
Albuterol		

16. Why are two antibiotics ordered for Sally Begay? How do they differ? What are the specific indications for both of these antibiotics?

17. Make a list of the routine medications you will be administering during the day shift at each of the following times.

Time	Medications to Be Given
0900	
1200	
1400	

18. A change in the medication orders is documented on Sally Begay's MAR for today. Did you see this change in order? What change occurred? Where can you verify this change in order? Do you need to change the information you recorded in question 17?

19. The ceftizoxime is ordered to be given IVPB. Sally Begay has a primary intravenous infusion of D_5 1/2 NS. Is ceftizoxime compatible with this primary solution? How can you find out?

20. Since Sally Begay is capable of drinking fluids, why does she have an IV running at D_5 1/2 NS at 75 cc/hour?

Pneumonia—Part II

👓 **Reading Assignment:** Nursing Assessment: Respiratory System (Chapter 24)
Nursing Management: Lower Respiratory System (Chapter 26)
Patient: Sally Begay, Room 304

In this lesson, you will continue working with Sally Begay, a 58-year-old Navajo woman with pneumonia. *(Note: You should have completed Lesson 16 prior to beginning this lesson.)*

💿 CD-ROM Activity

Go to the Supervisor's Office and sign in to work with Sally Begay for the Tuesday 0700 shift. Proceed to the bulletin board in the Nurses' Station to determine where report is being given for this patient. Go to that location.

1. As you listen to the report on Sally Begay, complete the following report form.

Red Rock Canyon Medical Center
Report Notes

Patient: Room #

Age: Diagnosis:

Vital Signs:

O$_2$ Sat:

Pain:

Treatments:

Significant Assessment Findings:

IV Location/Date:

Identified Patient/Family Problems:

171

2. There were two errors in the report you heard. Compare your data in question 1 of this lesson with what you learned about Sally Begay in Lesson 16. What information given to you by the nurse is incorrect?

3. What is the significance of these errors in the report? Will they ultimately affect your nursing care? What should you do about these errors?

→ It is time to take the patient's vital signs. Go to Sally Begay's room and click on **Vital Signs**.

4. Collect a full set of measurements and record your findings below.

Heart rate:

Blood pressure:

Temperature:

Respiratory rate:

Oxygen saturation:

Pain:

5. What did you observe about the oxygen saturation procedure that could affect the accuracy of the measurement?

6. Consider the data you recorded in question 4. Which data are out of normal range? Is there any action you would consider taking? If so, explain.

→ It is now time to complete a physical examination. Click first on **Physical** and then on each of the three specific examination areas.

7. Record your data for each area of Sally Begay's physical examination below.

Physical Examination Area	Data
Head and Neck	
Chest/Upper Extremities	
Abdomen and Lower Extremities	

8. What findings collected from the physical examination are useful in evaluating Sally Begay's status in regards to the pneumonia? What additional data would you have also included, based on what you observed during the examination?

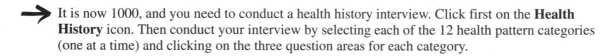

It is now 1000, and you need to conduct a health history interview. Click first on the **Health History** icon. Then conduct your interview by selecting each of the 12 health pattern categories (one at a time) and clicking on the three question areas for each category.

9. Record *significant data* from Sally Begay's health history below and on the next pages.

Health History Area	Data
Perception/Self-Concept	

Activity

Health History Area	Data
Sexuality/Reproduction	
Culture	
Nutrition-Metabolic	
Sleep-Rest	

Health History Area	Data
Role/Relationship	
Health Perception	
Elimination	
Cognitive/Perceptual	

Health History Area	Data
Coping/Stress	
Value/Belief	

10. Compare Sally Begay's presenting symptoms and her physical findings with the nursing assessment data commonly associated with pneumonia, as presented in the table below (Table 26-6 from your textbook). Circle or highlight data that are similar to findings for Sally Begay.

Subjective Data
Important Health Information
Past health history: Lung cancer, COPD, diabetes, chronic debilitating disease, malnutrition, altered consciousness, AIDS, exposure to chemical toxins, dust, or allergens
Medications: Use of antibiotics; corticosteroids, chemotherapy, or any other immunosuppressants
Surgeries or other treatment: Recent abdominal or thoracic surgery, splenectomy, endotracheal intubation, or any surgery with general anesthesia

Functional Health Patterns
Health perception-health management: Cigarette smoking, alcoholism; recent upper respiratory tract infection, malaise
Nutritional-metabolic: Anorexia, nausea, vomiting; chills
Activity-exercise: Prolonged bed rest or immobility; fatigue, weakness; dyspnea, cough (productive or nonproductive); nasal congestion
Cognitive-perceptual: Pain with breathing, chest pain, sore throat, headache, abdominal pain, muscle aches

Objective Data
General
Fever, restlessness or lethargy; splinting of affected area

Respiratory
Tachypnea; pharyngitis; asymmetric chest movements or retraction; decreased excursion; nasal flaring; use of accessory muscles (neck, abdomen); grunting; crackles, friction rub on auscultation; dullness on percussion over consolidated areas, increased tactile fremitus on palpation; pink, rusty, purulent, green, yellow, or white sputum (amount may be scant to copious)

Cardiovascular
Tachycardia

Neurologic
Changes in mental status, ranging from confusion to delirium

Possible Findings
Leukocytosis; abnormal ABGs with decreased or normal PaO_2, decreased $PaCO_2$, and increased pH initially, and later decreased PaO_2, increased $PaCO_2$, and decreased pH; positive sputum Gram's stain and culture; patchy or diffuse infiltrates, abscesses, pleural effusion, or pneumothorax on chest x-ray

11. Based on the health history interview, physical examination findings, and data from the chart, develop a list of nursing diagnoses and a list of collaborative problems for Sally Begay. Be sure that everything on your lists can be supported with data. *(Note: Refer to the care plan in your textbook for additional help.)*

Nursing Diagnoses   **Collaborative Problems**

12. Review the lists you developed in question 11. Choose two nursing diagnoses or collaborative problems *not found* on the care plan in the textbook. Develop these further by identifying patient outcomes and nursing interventions specific to Sally Begay's situation. Why did you select the ones that *you* did?

Nursing Diagnosis or Collaborative Problem	Outcomes	Nursing Interventions

→ Your next task is to do some follow-up regarding Sally Begay's condition. To accomplish this we are going to take a "virtual leap in time" to Friday morning. Go back to the Supervisor's Office and sign in again. (Remember: You will have to click on **Reset** before you can switch shifts.) Keep Sally Begay as your patient, but change your duty time to Friday 1100. Although Sally Begay was discharged home earlier this morning, her chart remains. Go to the Nurses' Station and open her chart.

13. Open the physicians' notes and read the notes from Tuesday until discharge. What changes occurred during the rest of the week?

14. Now read the nurses' notes. What changes in Sally Begay's status are evident through the documentation in the nurses' notes?

Review the pneumonia clinical pathway in your textbook.

15. What is the target length of stay for the pneumonia clinical pathway?

16. How many days was Sally Begay hospitalized?

17. If the nursing staff at Red Rock Canyon Medical Center had been using the textbook's clinical pathway, at what point (which day) would Sally Begay have significantly deviated from the pathway? If needed, go back to the chart to review the nurses' notes and compare these with the goals for the various days on the pathway.

18. What factor, more than any other, do you think was responsible for the extended hospital stay?

COPD

/ORO **Reading Assignment:** Nursing Assessment: Respiratory System (Chapter 24)
Nursing Management: Obstructive Pulmonary Disease
(Chapter 27)

Patient: Sally Begay, Room 304

You have been assigned to care for Sally Begay, a 58-year-old Navajo woman with a diagnosis of pneumonia. This patient also has a long-standing history of bronchitis. If you have already completed Lessons 16 and 17, you may want to refer back to some of the data you collected as you complete this lesson.

CD-ROM Activity

Go to the Supervisor's Office and sign in to work with Sally Begay for the Tuesday 0700 shift. Proceed to the Nurses' Station and open the patient's chart. In the Physical & History, read the admitting history completed in the Emergency Department at 1200. Next, close the chart and open Sally Begay's EPR. Read the entire Admissions Profile, which includes the nursing admission database.

1. How long has Sally Begay had bronchitis?

2. In addition to COPD and pneumonia, what other medical diagnoses does Sally Begay have?

3. Below, record the medications Sally Begay currently takes at home on a regular basis. Include the dosage and classification of each drug, as well as the reason the drug is taken.

Medication	Dose	Classification of Medication and Reason Taken

4. Based on her own medical history and her family history, what problem(s) is Sally Begay at risk for developing? Why?

In your textbook read the section on Emphysema and Chronic Bronchitis; then answer the following questions.

5. Define these terms: *chronic obstructive pulmonary disease*, *chronic bronchitis*, and *emphysema*.

Chronic obstructive pulmonary disease:

Chronic bronchitis:

Emphysema:

6. The textbook describes five major causes or etiologies of COPD. Below, identify those five etiologies, describe how each of these can lead to COPD, and indicate whether each etiology may have been a cause of chronic bronchitis for Sally Begay.

Etiology	Description of How This Can Lead to COPD

7. Based on the history in the patient's chart, which etiology or combination of etiologies seems most likely to have contributed to Sally Begay's COPD?

8. Briefly describe the pathophysiologic process of chronic bronchitis.

9. Draw a diagram of the pathophysiology of bronchitis.

10. What is the relationship between Sally Begay's primary admitting diagnosis (pneumonia) and the underlying chronic condition (chronic bronchitis)?

➤ Return to Sally Begay's chart, click on **Diagnostics**, and read the radiologic report by Dr. Kawasaka.

11. What findings on the CXR are consistent with COPD?

➤ Now flip back to the Physical & History. (Use the **Flip Back** icon in the lower right side of screen).

12. What was Sally Begay's arterial oxygen saturation in the Emergency Department? What is the normal range for oxygen saturation?

Sally Begay's O$_2$ Sat   **Normal Range O$_2$ Sat**

13. What exactly does an arterial oxygen saturation reflect? Why do you think her oxygen saturation deviates from normal?

→ Click on **Physicians' Orders**. Review the initial orders for Sally Begay written on Sunday night.

14. The physician ordered oxygen therapy. What was the order? What percentage of oxygen does this deliver?

15. What is the rationale for this oxygen order as opposed to high-flow oxygen administration to relieve the hypoxia?

16. Which of the medications listed is specific for treatment of COPD? What is the action of this drug? Describe how it is administered.

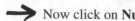 Now click on **Nurses' Notes** and read the notes for Saturday.

17. What problems have been identified by the nurse? What interventions have been planned? How do you think the effectiveness of these interventions will be evaluated? Record your answers below.

Identified Problems	Planned Interventions	How will these be evaluated?

18. Compare the identified problems and the planned interventions in the nurses' notes with the Nursing Care Plan in your textbook. What additional problems do you think should be included, based on what you know about Sally Begay?

→ Close Sally Begay's chart. Go to the computer under the bookshelf and access the EPR. Open Sally Begay's EPR and click on **Assessment**.

19. Compare the nursing assessment findings for Saturday at 1600 with those on Tuesday at 0400. Record your findings below.

Assessment Areas	Saturday 1600	Tuesday 0400
Temperature		
Heart rate		
Respiration		
Oxygen saturation		
Use of oxygen		
Respiratory pattern		
Lung fields		
Cough		
Sputum		

20. Based on the above assessment findings, how successful do you think the nursing interventions have been up to this point? What additional information would you want to consider?

21. What further interventions might be helpful in Sally Begay's case?

➡ Now we are going to move forward in time to Thursday. Return to the Supervisor's Office to sign in again. Keep Sally Begay as your patient, but change your duty time to Thursday 1100.

22. By Thursday afternoon Sally Begay is getting ready for discharge. Go to the Nurses' Station and find the location of the health team meeting. Attend the meeting and take notes as you listen.

Reporting	Important Data

Rose Simpson, RN
Nurse Case Manager

Louise Johnson, RN
Clinical Nurse Specialist

Kris Holmes, MSW
Social Worker

23. Consider the health team report you just heard. Now compare your notes with the Ambulatory and Home Care section in the textbook. Review Table 27-23 (Patient and Family Teaching Guide) as well. Were the discharge concerns for Sally Begay consistent with the textbook information? Is there anything else you would want to include in your discharge planning for this patient?

LESSON **19** —————————————————————————

Hypertension

————————————————————————————————————

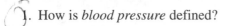 **Reading Assignment:** Nursing Assessment: Cardiovascular System (Chapter 30)
Nursing Management: Hypertension (Chapter 31)
Patient: Sally Begay, Room 304

Sally Begay is a 58-year-old Navajo woman with a diagnosis of pneumonia and chronic bronchitis. She also has a history of hypertension and coronary artery disease and a myocardial infarction 5 years ago. You have been assigned to review this patient's chart to learn more about hypertension.

In your textbook, read the Normal Regulation of Blood Pressure section; then answer the following questions.

1. How is *blood pressure* defined?

817

2. Complete and interpret the following equation.

Arterial blood pressure = _____ + _____

Interpretation:

3. What factors affect blood pressure? In the diagram below, illustrate the relationship of the variables in the equation in question 3 by filling in the various system factors that affect cardiac output and systemic vascular resistance.

818
Fig 31.1

Cardiac Factors	**Sympathetic Nervous System Factors**

Local Regulation

$$\text{Blood Pressure} = \text{Cardiac Output} \times \text{SVR}$$

Renal Factors	**Humoral Factors**

4. What role do baroreceptors play in the regulation of blood pressure? Where are they located, and what do they do?

8/7 2nd para. rt.

CD-ROM Activity

Go to the Supervisor's Office and sign in to work with Sally Begay for the Thursday 1100 shift. Proceed to the Nurses' Station and open her chart. In the Physical & History, read the admitting history completed in the Emergency Department at 1200.

5. How long has Sally Begay had a history of hypertension?

6. What was her admitting blood pressure in the Emergency Department?

7. What medications does Sally Begay currently take at home to treat her hypertension? Include the dosage and classification of the medication.

Medication	Dose	Classification of Medication

8. According to the textbook, how is *hypertension* defined? Before hypertension can be considered a true diagnosis, what conditions must exist?

9. What symptoms do you suspect Sally Begay experiences when her blood pressure is elevated?

10. If the blood pressure measurement recorded in the Emergency Department was reflective of Sally Begay's typical blood pressure without treatment, what stage of hypertension would she be experiencing?

→ Close Sally Begay's chart and open her EPR. Click on **Admissions** and read her entire Admissions Profile.

11. Based on the admission data and the data from the Emergency Department, what risk factors described in the textbook are present in Sally Begay's history? (Refer to Table 31-3 in the textbook for help.)

12. There are several important clues in the Admissions Profile that may provide insight into how Sally Begay manages her hypertension at home. What are they? What significance do they bear?

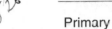

13. The textbook describes two general classifications of hypertension: primary and secondary. How are these differentiated?

Type of Hypertension	Description
Primary	
Secondary	

14. Do you suspect that Sally Begay has primary or secondary hypertension? Why?

15. There are many complications associated with hypertension. The textbook describes the most common complications in terms of target organ disease (TOD). These complications affect the heart, vessels, brain, kidney and eyes. Based on her history, does Sally Begay have evidence of current or previous TOD?

16. Consider the information presented in Table 31-7 (Risk Stratification and Treatment of Hypertension) in your textbook. In what risk group does Sally Begay belong, given the admitting blood pressure?

17. What is the purpose of risk stratification?

→ Close the EPR and return to the patient's chart. Click on **Physicians' Orders**.

18. Read the admission orders. Several diagnostic tests were ordered by the physician. Although these tests may have been ordered for various purposes, they might also help to identify the presence of other TOD. In the second column below, indicate how each test might be helpful. (Wait until questions 19 and 20 to fill in the third column.)

Diagnostic Test	How Test Might Help Identify TOD	Results
Chest x-ray		
BUN		
Creatinine		
ECG monitoring		

→ Now click on **Diagnostics** and read the chest x-ray report.

19. Record the results of the chest x-ray in the third column of the table in question 18 and indicate whether the results suggest the presence of TOD.

→ Close Sally Begay's chart and open her EPR.

20. Find and record the lab results for BUN, creatinine, and ECG monitoring in the table in question 18. Indicate what these results mean related to TOD.

Now click on **Vital Signs** and review the blood pressure trends for Sally Begay.

21. Record the blood pressure findings for the days and times listed below.

Day/Time	BP	Day/Time	BP
Saturday 1600		Tuesday 0800	
Saturday 2400		Tuesday 1600	
Sunday 0800		Tuesday 2400	
Sunday 1600		Wed 0800	
Sunday 2400		Wed 1600	
Monday 0800		Wed 2400	
Monday 1600		Thurs 0800	
Monday 2400		Thurs 1600	
		Thurs 2400	

22. What trend do you see in Sally Begay's vital signs? How can this be explained?

 23. Consider the treatment algorithm for hypertension in your textbook. Compare this with Sally Begay's case. In what way is Sally Begay's treatment not consistent with the textbook's drug choices, given her history and her BP trends noted in question 21?

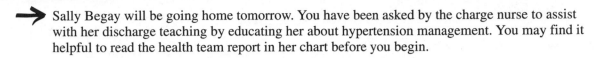 Sally Begay will be going home tomorrow. You have been asked by the charge nurse to assist with her discharge teaching by educating her about hypertension management. You may find it helpful to read the health team report in her chart before you begin.

24. Before you decide what to include in your patient teaching and how you are going to approach the teaching, what do you first need to assess?

25. Sally Begay tells you that she knows she has high blood pressure but does not really understand what it means or why it is harmful. She says she does not always take her medication and that sometimes she runs out. She also does not understand the need to monitor the blood pressure on a regular basis. Based on this data, develop a culturally appropriate teaching plan for Sally Begay.

Coronary Artery Disease

Reading Assignment: Nursing Assessment: Cardiovascular System (Chapter 30)
Nursing Management: Coronary Artery Disease (Chapter 32)
Patient: Sally Begay, Room 304

Sally Begay is a 58-year-old Navajo woman with a diagnosis of pneumonia and chronic bronchitis. She also has a history of hypertension and coronary artery disease, a myocardial infarction 5 years ago, and mild CHF. You have been assigned to review this patient's chart to learn more about coronary artery disease.

CD-ROM Activity

Go to the Supervisor's Office and sign in to work with Sally Begay for the Thursday 1100 shift. Proceed to the Nurses' Station and open her chart. In the Physical & History, read the admitting history completed in the Emergency Department at 1200.

1. Consider the risk factors for CAD. Identify each of the following risk factors as either unmodifiable (mark with a **U**) or modifiable (mark with an **M**). Circle those risk factors that are present in Sally Begay's history.

   _____ Age   _____ Family history

   _____ Elevated serum lipids   _____ Smoking

   _____ Inactivity   _____ Hypertension

   _____ Obesity   _____ Race

   _____ Gender   _____ Stress/behavior patterns

 In your textbook, read the Clinical Manifestations of Coronary Artery Disease section. The textbook describes three clinical manifestations of CAD: angina, myocardial infarction, and sudden cardiac death.

2. Sally Begay has intermittent angina. What is angina?

3. Describe what happens during an angina episode.

4. List at least five different factors that could precipitate myocardial ischemia and angina pain.

5. According to Sally Begay's history, how often does she have angina chest pain?

6. What medication does Sally Begay have at home in case she has angina? How does this drug work to treat angina?

7. Which of the three types of angina does Sally Begay most likely have? (Circle one.)

   Stable angina   Unstable angina   Prinzmetal's angina

8. Sally Begay had an MI 5 years ago. What is a myocardial infarction? Describe what happens during a myocardial infarction.

9. What is the relationship between having HTN and developing an MI?

10. What is the relationship between having an MI and developing CHF?

11. Read the Women and Coronary Artery Disease section in your textbook. Describe how this information is consistent with Sally Begay's history.

→ Click on **Physicians' Orders** in Sally Begay's chart. The physician has ordered ECG monitoring.

12. What does this mean? Why has this been ordered?

13. Based on this order, what should the nurses include in their documentation?

→ Now open the nurses' notes and read the notes for Saturday through Wednesday evening.

14. What do the nurses' notes reflect regarding the cardiac monitoring?

15. Nearly all of the nurses' notes indicate that Sally Begay says she has pain in her chest. How can the nurse differentiate chest pain from angina, chest pain from a myocardial infarction, and chest pain from pneumonia? (Refer to Table 32-9 in your textbook if you need help.)

→ You are asked by your nursing instructor to prepare patient teaching for Sally Begay. You decide to teach her about a healthy-heart diet as nutrition therapy education for coronary artery disease. First you need to collect pertinent data. Go into Sally Begay's room and click on **Health History**. Gather data in functional health pattern categories that you think will be helpful in your planning.

16. List pertinent data you collected from Sally Begay's health history interview that will help you plan your patient teaching.

17. What additional questions would you like to ask Sally Begay? What additional information would be helpful?

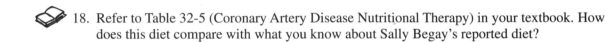

18. Refer to Table 32-5 (Coronary Artery Disease Nutritional Therapy) in your textbook. How does this diet compare with what you know about Sally Begay's reported diet?

19. Would Table 32-5 be appropriate to use as a guide to teach Sally Begay about CAD nutrition? Discuss some of the pros and cons of using this table.

LESSON 21

Congestive Heart Failure— Part I: Tuesday

✐ **Reading Assignment:** Nursing Management: Congestive Heart Failure and
Cardiac Surgery (Chapter 33)
Patient: Carmen Gonzales, Room 302

For this lesson, you have been assigned to care for Carmen Gonzales, a 56-year-old female admitted to the hospital with a severe leg infection. She also has a history of type 2 diabetes mellitus, coronary artery disease (CAD), congestive heart failure (CHF), and hypertension.

Before you begin, review the pathophysiologic factors associated with CHF.

1. CHF typically manifests as:
   a. right-sided failure.
   b. left-sided failure.
   c. biventricular failure.

2. The most common form of initial heart failure is:
   a. right-sided failure.
   b. left-sided failure.
   c. biventricular failure.

3. Compare and contrast the most common causes of right-sided CHF and left-sided CHF below.

Left-Sided Failure   **Right-Sided Failure**

4. On the figure below, complete the following activities:

   a. Illustrate normal blood flow through the heart. Draw arrows to represent flow.

   b. Illustrate afterload. Write the word *afterload* (to represent hypertension) next to the descending aorta.

   c. Illustrate the backup of fluid from the left side of the heart (left ventricle) into the pulmonary vein and into the lungs.

   d. Illustrate pulmonary edema by drawing dots or small circles on the lungs to show the location of excess fluid.

   e. Illustrate the backup of fluid from the pulmonary artery into the right side of the heart and then into the peripheral system (superior and inferior vena cava).

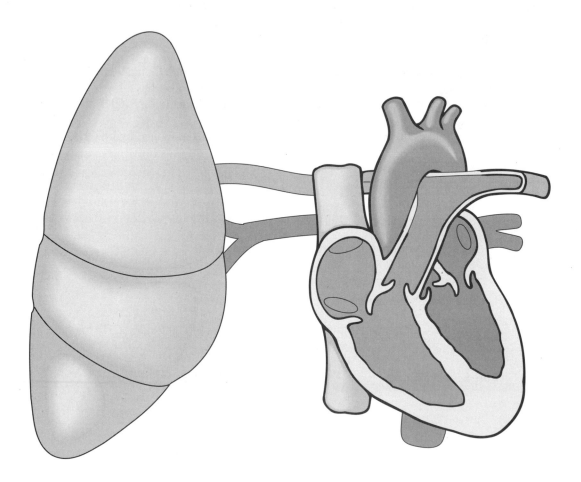

CD-ROM Activity

Go to the Supervisor's Office and sign in to work with Carmen Gonzales for the Tuesday 0700 shift. Go to the Nurses' Station and open her chart. Read the Physical & History, including the Emergency Department Record. (Remember to scroll down to read all pages.)

5. What information is found in the Physical & History that specifically addresses Carmen Gonzales and her CHF?

6. If you had done the initial ER assessment of Carmen Gonzales, what additional history or examination would you have included specifically to assess the status of her CHF?

7. Your textbook identifies several risk factors for the development of CHF. Compare this information with the data found in Carmen Gonzales' chart. Below and on the next page, indicate whether Carmen Gonzales has each of the listed risk factors. Then record the data from the patient's chart that support your opinion.

Risk Factors	Does Carmen Gonzales have this risk factor?	What data support your answer?
Advancing age		
Coronary artery disease		
Hypertension		
Diabetes		

Risk Factors	Does Carmen Gonzales have this risk factor?	What data support your answer?
Smoking		
Obesity		
Elevated cholesterol levels		

→ Close Carmen Gonzales' chart. Access her EPR and read the Admissions Profile.

8. What data in the profile provide clues regarding the presence of symptoms of CHF?

→ Close the EPR and return to the patient's chart. Click on **Physicians' Orders** and review the orders for Carmen Gonzales.

9. What orders are present in Carmen Gonzales' chart that specifically address monitoring and management of her congestive heart failure?

→ The night nurse is ready to start report on Carmen Gonzales. Close the patient's chart and go to hear the report. (Remember: You can find out where report is being given by checking the bulletin board or by moving your cursor across the animated map.)

10. What did you think about the report you were given? Is there anything you wished the nurse would have included in the report regarding Carmen Gonzales' CHF? If so, what? The nurse in the report suggested you keep a close eye on the patient. How will you do this? What will you watch for? (Refer to Table 33-3 in your textbook for help.)

→ It is now 0745. Go inside Carmen Gonzales' room and click on **Vital Signs**.

11. Obtain a set of vital signs and record your findings below.

Temperature _____   Respiration _____

Heart rate _____   Blood pressure _____

Pain rating _____   Oxygen saturation _____

12. Consider the vital signs you just obtained. Are there any that concern you? If so, which one(s)?

→ Go to the Nurses' Station and access the EPR for Carmen Gonzales. Click on **Vital Signs**.

13. Review the vital sign data for Carmen Gonzales for the last couple of days and compare it with your findings in question 11. What would be the appropriate action by the nurse in this situation?

Return to Carmen Gonzales' room. Conduct a health history and physical examination, focusing particularly on data suggesting CHF.

14. The table below lists common assessment findings for CHF.

   a. Place an asterisk (*) next to any data in the table that you also collected during your assessment of Carmen Gonzales.

Table 21-1   Congestive Heart Failure

Subjective Data	Objective Data
Important Health Information	**Integumentary**
Past health history: CAD (including recent MI), hypertension, cardiomyopathy, valvular or congenital heart disease, diabetes mellitus, thyroid or lung disease, rapid or irregular heartbeat	Cool, diaphoretic skin; cyanosis or pallor, peripheral edema (right-sided heart failure)
Medications: Use of and compliance with any cardiac medications; use of diuretics, estrogens, corticosteroids, phenylbutazone, nonsteroidal antiinflammatory drugs	**Respiratory** Tachypnea, crackles, rhonchi, wheezes; frothy, blood-tinged sputum
	Cardiovascular
Functional Health Patterns	Tachycardia, S_3, S_4, murmurs; pulsus alternans, PMI displaced inferiorly and posteriorly, jugular vein distention
Health perception-health management: Fatigue	
Nutritional-metabolic: Usual sodium intake; nausea, vomiting, anorexia, stomach bloating; weight gain	**Gastrointestinal** Abdominal distention, hepatosplenomegaly, ascites
Elimination: Nocturia, decreased daytime urinary output, constipation	
Activity-exercise: Dyspnea, orthopnea, cough; palpitations; dizziness, fainting	**Neurologic** Restlessness, confusion, decreased attention or memory
Sleep-rest: Number of pillows used for sleeping; paroxysmal nocturnal dyspnea	
Cognitive-perceptual: Chest pain or heaviness; RUQ pain, abdominal discomfort; behavioral changes	**Possible Findings** Altered serum electrolytes (especially Na^+ and K^+), elevated BUN, creatinine, or liver function tests; chest x-ray demonstrating cardiomegaly, pulmonary congestion, and interstitial pulmonary edema; echocardiogram showing increased chamber size and decreased wall motion; atrial and ventricular enlargement on ECG; ↑ PAP, ↑ PAWP, ↓ CO, ↓ CI, ↓ O_2 saturation, ↑ SVR on hemodynamic monitoring

   b. For each finding you marked, briefly explain what led you to this decision.

15. Based on what you have assessed, identify from the following list the most significant priorities for Carmen Gonzales for the rest of your shift. (Place an **X** next to all diagnoses or collaborative problems that apply at this time.)

_____ Pain   _____ Risk for impaired gas exchange

_____ Risk for fall   _____ Ineffective management of therapeutic regime

_____ Activity intolerance   _____ Impaired skin integrity

_____ Fluid volume depletion   _____ Risk for altered role performance

_____ PC: Pulmonary edema   _____ PC: Increased intracranial pressure

Congestive Heart Failure— Part II: Thursday

⌒∞ **Reading Assignment:** Nursing Management: Congestive Heart Failure and
Cardiac Surgery (Chapter 33)
Patient: Carmen Gonzales, Room 302

For this lesson, you will continue your assignment for Carmen Gonzales, a 56-year-old female admitted to the hospital with a severe leg infection. She also has a history of type 2 DM, coronary artery disease (CAD), congestive heart failure (CHF), and hypertension. You should complete Lesson 21 prior to beginning this lesson.

CD-ROM Activity

Go to the Supervisor's Office and sign in to work with Carmen Gonzales for the Thursday 0700 shift. Before you visit your patient, go to the Nurses' Station and review her chart to determine changes in her status since you cared for her on Tuesday. Click on **Nurses' Notes** and read the notes for Tuesday afternoon and Wednesday.

1. Now that you have read the nurses' notes in Carmen Gonzales' chart, list below any significant data you found regarding CHF.

2. Now read the physicians' orders. Record the orders for Tuesday afternoon below.

221

→ Next, click on **Diagnostics** in Carmen Gonzales' chart.

3. Read and record the radiology report for Tuesday afternoon.

4. Read the cardiology consultation for Tuesday and Wednesday. What do these findings show?

5. According to her chart, Carmen Gonzales had a short episode of right-sided CHF caused by fluid volume overload after you left the hospital on Tuesday afternoon. What specific signs and symptoms did she have that are consistent with a diagnosis of right-sided heart failure? On the table below, put an asterisk (*) next to any data you collected from the cardiology report, radiology report, or nurses' notes in the patient's chart.

Subjective Data
Important Health Information
Past health history: CAD (including recent MI), hypertension, cardiomyopathy, valvular or congenital heart disease, diabetes mellitus, thyroid or lung disease, rapid or irregular heartbeat
Medications: Use of and compliance with any cardiac medications; use of diuretics, estrogens, corticosteroids, phenylbutazone, nonsteroidal antiinflammatory drugs

Functional Health Patterns
Health perception-health management: Fatigue
Nutritional-metabolic: Usual sodium intake; nausea, vomiting, anorexia, stomach bloating; weight gain
Elimination: Nocturia, decreased daytime urinary output, constipation
Activity-exercise: Dyspnea, orthopnea, cough; palpitations; dizziness, fainting
Sleep-rest: Number of pillows used for sleeping; paroxysmal nocturnal dyspnea
Cognitive-perceptual: Chest pain or heaviness; RUQ pain, abdominal discomfort; behavioral changes

Objective Data
Integumentary
Cool, diaphoretic skin; cyanosis or pallor, peripheral edema (right-sided heart failure)

Respiratory
Tachypnea, crackles, rhonchi, wheezes; frothy, blood-tinged sputum

Cardiovascular
Tachycardia, S_3, S_4, murmurs; pulsus alternans, PMI displaced inferiorly and posteriorly, jugular vein distention

Gastrointestinal
Abdominal distention, hepatosplenomegaly, ascites

Neurologic
Restlessness, confusion, decreased attention or memory

Possible Findings
Altered serum electrolytes (especially Na^+ and K^+), elevated BUN, creatinine, or liver function tests; chest x-ray demonstrating cardiomegaly, pulmonary congestion, and interstitial pulmonary edema; echocardiogram showing increased chamber size and decreased wall motion; atrial and ventricular enlargement on ECG; ↑ PAP, ↑ PAWP, ↓ CO, ↓ CI, ↓ O_2 saturation, ↑ SVR on hemodynamic monitoring

Close the chart and access the EPR for Carmen Gonzales. Click on **I&O**.

6. Review the intake and output records since Carmen Gonzales' admission. Calculate the following information:

	Total Intake	**Total Output**
Sunday		
Monday		
Tuesday through 1500		
3-day totals		

7. What conclusions can be made regarding the findings recorded in question 6?

8. Explain the signs and symptoms Carmen Gonzales has experienced from a pathophysiologic perspective. How did fluid volume overload cause her symptoms?

As you know, the physician ordered furosemide 20 mg IV stat on Tuesday afternoon. Use a nursing drug reference to answer the following questions.

9. What is the action of furosemide? (In other words, how does it work, and on what part of the kidney does its action take place?)

10. What is the desired therapeutic effect of furosemide? How could the nurse assess whether this desired effect was achieved?

11. Why would furosemide be the diuretic of choice to use in this situation, as opposed to a thiazide diuretic? Why was it given IV instead of orally?

12. Refer again to the intake and output record in the EPR. What happened to the urine output after the furosemide was administered? Now calculate the 24-hour I&O totals for Sunday through Wednesday.

	Total Intake	**Total Output**
Sunday		
Monday		
Tuesday		
Wednesday		
3-day totals		

13. What conclusions can be made regarding the data you recorded in question 12?

→ Close the EPR notes and open Carmen Gonzales' MAR (in the blue notebook on the counter).

14. Determine what routine medications you will be giving to Carmen Gonzales today during your shift (0700 to 1500). Below, list the medication(s) you need to give and the time each is due.

Medication	Why Given	Time Due

15. Now find out where the night nurse is giving report on Carmen Gonzales. Go to that location and listen to report. Record any pertinent information below.

16. Did you notice any discrepancies in the report from what you read in the chart? If so, explain.

→ It is now 0745. Go to Carmen Gonzales' room and click on **Vital Signs**.

17. Obtain a set of vital signs and record your findings below.

Temperature _____   Respiration _____

Heart rate _____   Blood pressure _____

Pain rating _____   Oxygen saturation _____

→ Go to the Nurses' Station and open the EPR for Carmen Gonzales. Record the vital signs. Close the EPR.

It is 0800. Return to Carmen Gonzales' room. Click on **Medications** and administer the 0800 medications to the patient.

Your nursing instructor suggests that you participate in Carmen Gonzales' discharge planning and patient teaching. To prepare for this, do the following:

- Go to the discharge planning meeting today (see the bulletin board in the Nurses' Station for location.)
- Review the Physical & History and the health team reports in the patient's chart.
- Consider the data you collected during your interview and examination on Tuesday (review these again if needed).
- Review the data in the Admissions Profile in Carmen Gonzales' EPR.

18. What specific issues have you identified from Carmen Gonzales' data that may influence how you approach her discharge teaching?

19. How does Carmen Gonzales' ethnicity factor into her discharge teaching?

→ Your instructor suggests that you briefly teach Carmen Gonzales about low-sodium diets. (The dietitian will spend time with her prior to discharge specifically to develop a menu plan with her that addresses DM and CHF.) You decide to go over four points about low-sodium diets.

20. Using Table 33-10 and Table 33-11 from your textbook, complete the following teaching instruction sheet for Carmen Gonzales.

- What is a low-sodium diet?

- Why is a low-sodium diet important for you to follow?

- Many of the foods that you currently enjoy can be included on this diet. They are:

- There are several foods that should be avoided, if possible, on this diet. Examples include:

After teaching Carmen Gonzales about the low-sodium diet, your instructor suggests that you review the CHF Patient and Family Teaching Guide with her (Table 33-13 in your textbook).

21. In what way would you tailor the CHF teaching guide to meet Carmen Gonzales' needs?

LESSON **23** ————————————————————————

Nutritional Problems

————————————————————————————————————

/⊙乃 **Reading Assignment:** Nursing Management: Nutritional Problems (Chapter 38)
Patient: Ira Bradley, Room 309

For this lesson, you will apply nutrition concepts to the case of Ira Bradley. Ira is a 43-year-old male admitted to the hospital with a diagnosis of late-state HIV infection, *Pneumocystis carinii* pneumonia, candidiasis, and Kaposi's sarcoma.

🔘 **CD-ROM Aotivity**

Go to the Supervisor's Office and sign in to work with Ira Bradley for the Thursday 0700 shift. Proceed to the Nurses' Station and open his chart. Read the Emergency Department Report in the Physical & History.

1. What problems related to nutrition are evident by reading the Emergency Department Report?

 2. According to the textbook, why do conditions such as HIV infection contribute to weight loss?

Several anthropometric measurements are useful in evaluating nutritional status.

3. Look again at the Emergency Department Report for Ira Bradley. What are his admission height and weight?

Height _____

Weight _____

4. What is body mass index (BMI)? What is the normal or ideal, BMI range?

5. Determine Ira Bradley's BMI using the nomogram in your textbook.

BMI = _____

6. What does Ira Bradley's BMI reflect?

Biochemical or laboratory tests are also helpful in evaluation of nutritional status. In Ira Bradley's chart, review the initial physicians' orders written on Sunday night.

7. What laboratory test was done that is helpful to understand the patient's current status?

8. Compare Ira Bradley's admission albumin level with the normal range as given in Table 38-12 in your textbook.

Ira Bradley's level _____

Normal range _____

9. What does Ira Bradley's lab value indicate?

10. What is the difference between albumin and prealbumin levels?

 It should be obvious to you by now that Ira Bradley suffers from malnutrition. Refer to the textbook and read about nutritional needs of patients with physical illness.

11. According to your textbook, how does fever affect metabolic rate and nutritional needs?

→ 12. Close the patient's chart and open the EPR. Click on **Vital Signs**; then record Ira Bradley's temperature for the first 24 hours after admission.

Sunday 2400 _____   Monday 1200 _____

Monday 0400 _____   Monday 1600 _____

Monday 0800 _____   Monday 2000 _____

13. How much of an increase in BMR would you estimate Ira Bradley experienced the first 24 hours?

Clearly, a goal of nursing care for Ira Bradley's is to improve his nutritional status. Let's evaluate his nutritional intake during this hospitalization.

→ 14. How many calories do you think Ira Bradley took in between admission and Tuesday morning (before breakfast)? You won't find this specific information on the chart, but you can make an educated guess by completing the following steps:

a. An IV fluid was ordered for Ira Bradley upon admission. What specifically was the order? (If you don't remember, go back to his chart and review the physicians' orders.)

b. How many calories are in 1 liter of the IV fluid he received? (You may have to look in other sources for this information.)

c. Go back to the EPR and click on **I&0**. Approximately how much IV fluid did Ira Bradley receive during the first 24 hours since admission (Sunday 2400 to Monday 2400)?

d. Approximately how many total calories did Ira Bradley receive from the IV fluid? Record this in the chart below.

e. What meal(s) did Ira Bradley eat during the first 24 hours since admission? What percentage of his meal(s) did he intake during that time? (In the EPR, click on **ADL**, then on **Appetite**.) What is your best guess of total calories he consumed in the meal(s)? Record this in the chart below.

f. What would you estimate as Ira Bradley's total caloric intake between Sunday 2400 and Tuesday 0800? Record this below.

g. What would you guess Ira Bradley's caloric requirements are per day? Refer to Table 38-5 in the textbook to help you estimate this. Record this below.

h. Now calculate the net difference between Ira Bradley's caloric needs and his actual intake during this time. Record this below.

Total calories from IV   _____

Estimated calories from   _____
meals (not including
Tuesday's breakfast)

Estimated caloric intake   _____
(Sunday 2400–
Tuesday 0800)

Estimated caloric needs   _____
per 24 hours

Net difference between   _____
caloric needs and
actual intake

15. What is your assessment of Ira Bradley's intake as recorded in question 14?

16. Review Ira Bradley's eating patterns for the rest of the week. What pattern of intake do you see, based on documentation in the EPR?

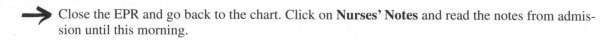 Close the EPR and go back to the chart. Click on **Nurses' Notes** and read the notes from admission until this morning.

17. Do the nurses' notes address Ira Bradley's nutritional status adequately? Explain.

 18. Review the various types of supplemental nutrition (tube feedings and parenteral nutrition) described in your textbook. Should any of these measures have been implemented?

19. What suggestions might you make to Ira Bradley and his wife regarding improvement of his nutritional status once he goes home?

LESSON **24** ——————————————————

Diabetes Mellitus—
Part I: Tuesday

——————————————————————————

 Reading Assignment: Nursing Assessment: Endocrine System (Chapter 45)
Nursing Management: Patient with Diabetes Mellitus
(Chapter 46)
Patient: Carmen Gonzales, Room 302

For this lesson, you are assigned to care for Carmen Gonzales, a 56-year-old female patient admitted to the hospital with type 2 diabetes mellitus and a leg infection.

Before you begin, review the pathophysiologic factors associated with type 2 diabetes mellitus (DM) in your textbook.

1. What three factors associated with type 2 DM result in peripheral insulin resistance?

2. Complete the following chart, comparing and contrasting the characteristics of type 1 and type 2 diabetes mellitus.

Characteristics	Type 1 Diabetes Mellitus	Type 2 Diabetes Mellitus
Age of onset		
Causes		
Symptoms at onset		
Use of insulin		
Use of oral hypoglycemic agents		
Common complications		

CD-ROM Activity

Go to the Supervisor's Office and sign in to work with Carmen Gonzales for the Tuesday 0700 shift. Before you visit the patient, go to the Nurses' Station and briefly review parts of her chart. Read the entire History & Physical, including the Emergency Department Record (Remember to scroll down to read all pages.)

3. What data in the chart specifically addresses Carmen Gonzales and her diabetes?

4. If you had done the initial ER assessment of Carmen Gonzales, what additional history or examination would you have included?

5. According to her medical history, Carmen Gonzales has coronary artery disease, hypertension, and congestive heart failure, and she had a severe right leg infection within the last 5 months. Is there a relationship between her diabetes and these other problems? If so, what might they be? Record your answers below and on the next page.

Medical Diagnosis	Relationship to Type 2 Diabetes Mellitus
Coronary artery disease	
Hypertension	

Medical Diagnosis	Relationship to Type 2 Diabetes Mellitus
Congestive heart failure	
Infection to leg	

6. The textbook describes the clinical picture of type 2 diabetes mellitus. Fill in the following chart, comparing data from the textbook with data found in the Carmen Gonzales' Physical & History. Does she fit the clinical picture?

Clinical Picture	Textbook Description	Carmen Gonzales' Data	Fits Description? (Yes or No)
Age of onset			
Ethnicity			
Obesity			
Familial factors			

→ Click on **Physicians' Orders** and review the orders for Carmen Gonzales.

7. What orders are present that specifically address management of her diabetes?

→ Now click on **Expired MARs** and review this data.

8. How many times has insulin been given to Carmen Gonzales? At what dose(s)?

9. Carmen Gonzales does not take insulin at home. Why has it been ordered for this hospitalization? Why does she suddenly need it now?

10. As part of your clinical preparation, research information about glyburide in your textbook or your drug reference. Complete the following drug card based on your research.

DRUG CARD

Generic Name: Glyburide

Common Trade Names:

Mechanism of Action:

Dosage:

Administration Routes:

➡ Close the patient's chart and access Carmen Gonzales' current MAR (in the blue notebook on the counter).

11. Determine what routine medications you will be administering to Carmen Gonzales today during the day shift (0700–1500). Below, list the routine medication(s) you need to give her, the reason why the med(s) will be given, and the time the med(s) should be given.

Medication	Why Given	Time Due

→ The nurse from the previous shift is ready to give report on Carmen Gonzales. Close the MAR, find out where report is being given, and go to hear report.

12. What did you think about the report you were given? Is there anything you wished the nurse would have included in the report regarding the patient's DM? If so, what?

→ It is now 0745. Go inside Carmen Gonzales' room and click on **Vital Signs**. Obtain a set of vital signs, and record your findings in the EPR. (You will need to leave the patient's room and go to one of the computers that access the EPR.)

13. Based on what you learned from obtaining vital signs, you should return to Carmen Gonzales' room and administer a PRN medication. What medication is appropriate? Why?

→ It is now time to give Carmen Gonzales her 0800 medications. Return to her room and click on **Medications** to complete this activity.

14. Consider administration guidelines associated with administration of glyburide. What is the rationale for administering glyburide at 0800? (You may need to refer to your nursing drug book.)

15. You learn from the charge nurse that Carmen Gonzales was given 6 units of regular SQ at 0730 (while you were listening to report) for a blood sugar of 260. Refer to your drug book or the textbook, and fill in the following information regarding regular insulin.

	Expected Length of Time	Actual Time After 0730 Dose
Onset		
Peak		
Duration		

→ You are now ready to conduct a physical examination of Carmen Gonzales. Click on **Physical** and obtain data in the three assessment areas.

16. Record your physical examination findings below and on the next page. Then go to the EPR and record the findings there as well.

Assessment	Finding
Head and Neck	
Chest/Upper Extremities	

Assessment	Finding
Abdomen and Lower Extremities	

17. Do any of your findings deviate from what you expected?

25

Diabetes Mellitus—
Part II: Thursday

/ORO **Reading Assignment:** Nursing Assessment: Patient With Diabetes Mellitus (Chapter 46)
Patient: Carmen Gonzales, Room 302

For this lesson, you will continue to care for Carmen Gonzales, a 56-year-old female patient admitted to the hospital with type 2 diabetes mellitus and a leg infection. You should complete Lesson 24 before beginning this lesson.

CD-ROM Activity

Go to the Supervisor's Office and sign in to work with Carmen Gonzales for the Thursday 0700 shift. Proceed to the Nurses' Station and open the patient's chart. Briefly review parts of the chart to update you regarding her care since Tuesday. Specifically, review the expired MARs, physicians' notes, physicians' orders, and nurses' notes. When you are finished, close the chart and access Carmen Gonzales' MAR. Determine what routine medications you will be giving to Carmen Gonzales today during the day shift (0700–1500).

1. Below, list the routine medication(s) you need to give this patient. Also explain why you need to give the med(s) and record the time you need to administer the med(s).

Medication	Why Given	Time Due

2. When and why did the physician order furosemide for Carmen Gonzales? What effect could it have related to her diabetes? (Refer to a nursing drug book or your textbook for help.)

The night nurse is ready to give report on Carmen Gonzales. Close the MAR and check the bulletin board for the location of the report. Go there and listen to report.

3. What did you think about the report you were given? Is there anything you wished the nurse would have included in the report regarding Carmen Gonzales' DM? If so, what?

4. It is almost 0800. Go into Carmen Gonzales' room and obtain a set of vital signs. Record your findings below and in the EPR.

Heart rate _____

Respiration _____

Blood pressure _____

Temperature _____

Oxygen saturation _____

Pain rating _____

→ Return to Carmen Gonzales' room and administer her 0800 medications.

Your nursing instructor has asked that you participate in Carmen Gonzales' discharge planning. Before you do this, you need to collect more data. In the patient's room, click on **Health History** and conduct a patient interview. Specifically, pay attention to information that would be helpful in developing a plan of care for her at discharge, focusing on the diabetes.

5. Below and on the next two pages, record the data you have collected from the health history interview that will help you as you develop a plan of care for Carmen Gonzales.

Health History Area	Data
Perception/Self-Concept	
Activity	
Sexuality/Reproductive	
Culture	
Nutrition-Metabolic	

Health History Area	Data
Sleep-Rest	
Role/Relationship	
Health Perception	
Elimination	
Cognitive/Perceptual	
Coping/Stress	

Health History Area	**Data**
Value/Belief	

6. What specific issues have you identified from Carmen Gonzales' medical history, interview, and assessment that may influence how you go about discharge teaching for diabetes management?

7. How does your cultural assessment of Carmen Gonzales factor into your discharge teaching?

8. After considering the subjective and objective data for Carmen Gonzales, develop a list of nursing diagnoses and collaborative problems below. Include goals and possible interventions for each diagnosis or problem. Compare your problem list with the Nursing Care Plan for Home and Ambulatory Setting in the textbook. In what way does this plan of care relate to Carmen Gonzales' needs? What adaptations need to be made?

Nursing Diagnosis or Collaborative Problem	Goals	Interventions

→ Go to the discharge planning meeting today (see the bulletin board in the Nurses' Station for location). Also, read the health team reports in Carmen Gonzales' chart.

9. What types of needs does Carmen Gonzales have for dietary management related to her type 2 DM?

10. Below is a diagram representing the general dietary strategy for patients with type 2 diabetes. Using data you have gathered from Carmen Gonzales and information from your textbook, make specific suggestions to the patient related to each of the boxes in the diagram. Write your ideas directly on the diagram.

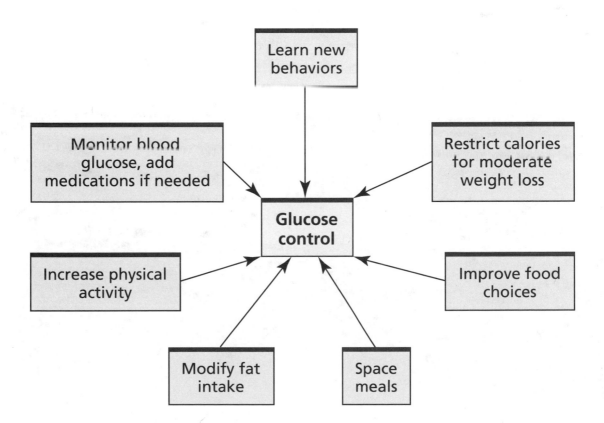

LESSON **26** ————————————————————————

Closed Head Injury

———

/OᴼᴼᴼᴼᴼᴼᴼD **Reading Assignment:** Nursing Assessment: Neurologic System (Chapter 53)
Nursing Management: Intracranial Problems (Chapter 54)
Patient: David Ruskin, Room 303

For this lesson, you will study the case of David Ruskin, a 31-year-old male admitted to the hospital following a bicycle accident. He has been diagnosed with a closed head injury, fractured right humerus, and scalp laceration.

CD-ROM Activity

Go to the Supervisor's Office and sign in to work with David Ruskin for the Tuesday 0700 shift. Proceed to the Nurses' Station and open his chart. Read the Emergency Department (ED) Report in the Physical & History section.

1. According to the Emergency Department Report, what was the mechanism of injury for David Ruskin? What other data are important to note regarding the accident and events immediately after the accident?

2. What was David Ruskin's neurologic status upon arrival to the ED?

255

3. What is the Glasgow Coma Scale? What are the three components of this scale? What does David Ruskin's score mean?

1609

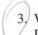

Following a head injury, the physician's initial concern is cerebral edema and increased intracranial pressure (ICP). Answer the following questions related to these concepts. Refer to your textbook for help, if necessary.

4. What can cause cerebral edema following a head injury?

1613 Table 54-4

5. How does cerebral edema lead to ICP? What is the mechanism of increased ICP?

1613

*Vasogenic CE – As in endothelial lining of cere.
capillaries allow leckage of macromolecules
from caps into surrounding extracellular space.
this*

6. An immediate action by the Emergency Department staff was to administer high-flow oxygen to David Ruskin. Why was this done?

Review the content in the textbook regarding complications of head injury.

7. If David Ruskin has suffered a severe head injury resulting in increased ICP, what symptoms should you expect to see?

8. Two diagnostic tests were conducted in the Emergency Department to gain further information regarding David Ruskin's head injury: CT scan and skull series. What is the difference between these two tests? Why were these ordered?

Test	Description of Test and Reason Ordered
CT scan	
Skull series	

9. What were the results of the CT scan and skull series?

10. What is the main problem associated with CT scan for a patient who is not fully oriented? What can be done to help alleviate this problem?

→ Return to David Ruskin's chart and open the physicians' orders.

11. Read the postoperative orders for David Ruskin. Which orders specifically reflect the closed head injury diagnosis?

12. How are vital signs an important aspect of monitoring a patient with a closed head injury?

13. According to the physicians' orders, the nurses are to do "neuro checks." What should be included?

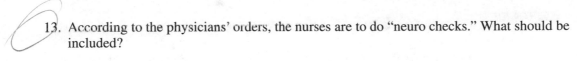 Now open the nurses' notes. Read the notes for Sunday and Monday.

14. What references are made in the documentation related to neurologic status?

Close the patient's chart and check the bulletin board to see where the night nurse is giving report on David Ruskin. Go to that location and listen to report.

15. What pertinent information related to David Ruskin's neurologic status is given in report?

16. What, if any, information did you find confusing during report? Is there anything else you would have liked the nurse to have included in the report? If so, what?

➤ Now go into David Ruskin's room, click on **Vital Signs**, and obtain a set of vital sign readings.

17. Record David Ruskin's vital sign readings below. Then go to one of the computers that allow you to access the EPR and record them there as well.

Temperature _____   Respiration _____

Blood pressure _____   Oxygen saturation _____

Heart rate _____   Pain rating _____

➤ Click on **Health History**, then on **Cognitive/Perceptual**, and listen to David Ruskin's responses in all three question areas. When you are finished, return to his chart in the Nurses' Station. Read through the Physical & History again, this time paying attention for data related to neurologic function.

18. Based on the data in these two areas, what can you document regarding the following neurologic findings?

Mental status

Pupil response/size

Glascow Coma Scale

Motor strength

Other cranial nerves assessed

19. It has been 36 hours since David Ruskin's injury. Based on your assessment findings, indicate for each of the following possible types of head injury whether you think it is likely or unlikely that David Ruskin has this type of injury.

Epidural hematoma:

Acute subdural hematoma:

Subacute subdural hematoma:

20. Based on your answer to question 19, explain why this type of injury is still possible and how you might assess for it.

Acute Spinal Cord Injury— Part I: Preclinical Preparation

Reading Assignment: Nursing Management: Peripheral Nerve and Spinal Cord Problems (Chapter 57)

Patient: Andrea Wang, Room 310

For this lesson, you will complete preclinical preparation for Andrea Wang, a 20-year-old female who was admitted to the hospital a week ago following an acute spinal cord injury. The day of the injury, the patient went to emergency surgery and spent a week in ICU. On Monday of this week, she was transferred to the medical-surgical unit.

CD-ROM Activity

Go to the Supervisor's Office and sign in to work with Andrea Wang for the Tuesday 0700 shift. Proceed to the Nurses' Station and open her chart. Read the entire Physical & History, including the Emergency Department Record. (Remember to scroll down to read all pages.)

1. According to the Emergency Department Record, what was the mechanism of injury for Andrea Wang?

2. What are Andrea Wang's initial neurologic examination findings?

Area	Findings
Pupils	
Glasgow Coma Scale	
Orientation	
Cranial nerves	
Peripheral nerves	

3. Several radiographic diagnostic studies were performed in the Emergency Department, including a chest x-ray and an MRI. According to the Emergency Department Record, what do these studies reveal?

Read about spinal cord trauma in your textbook.

4. Describe the pathophysiology of spinal cord trauma during the acute or initial injury stage.

5. Why is spinal edema such a serious concern following an acute spinal cord injury?

6. Which of the following pictures represents the type of spinal injury Andrea Wang has suffered? Circle the correct answer.

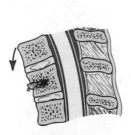

Flexion injury

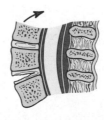

Extension injury

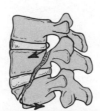

Flexion-rotation injury

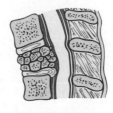

Compression injury

7. According to the Emergency Department Record, Andrea Wang has a partially transected spinal cord at T6. What does *partial transection* mean?

8. What are the four types of syndromes associated with a partial transection of the spinal cord?

   a.

   b.

   c.

   d.

9. Which of the four syndromes from question 8 do you suspect Andrea Wang is experiencing? Why?

10. The physician indicates that Andrea Wang also suffers from spinal shock. Describe spinal shock.

11. According to the Emergency Department Record, a Foley catheter was inserted in the Emergency Department. What, if anything, does this have to do with Andrea Wang's spinal cord injury?

12. The physician's plan also included "steroid protocol for spinal injury." What drug is typically used for this? What is the usual dose, and how is it given in this situation? What benefit does this provide? (You may need to refer to a drug handbook.)

Drug	Typical Dose and Administration	Beneficial Effects

13. Andrea Wang was sent to the OR for decompression and fusion of the thoracic spine within 1 1/2 hours of arrival. What is the purpose of this surgical procedure, and why was it done immediately?

→ In Andrea Wang's chart, click on **Physicians' Orders** and review the orders for Monday (*not including medication orders*).

14. Indicate the rationale for the physician's orders. (If you need help, consult the Care Plan in your textbook.)

Orders (not including medications)	Rationale

➡ Close Andrea Wang's chart and open the MAR (in the blue notebook on the counter).

15. Examine the list of medications Andrea Wang is receiving. Why are they being given?

Medication	Classification	Reason Given
Famotidine 20 mg PO q12h		
Docusate sodium 100 mg PO qd		
Biscodyl suppository 10 mg, QOD PRN		
Multiple vitamin with minerals qAM		
Vitamin C 500 mg PO qPM		
Enoxaparin 30 mg SC q12h		
Baclofen 10 mg PO q12h		
Acetaminophen 600 mg PO q4–6h PRN		
Oxycodone/ acetominophen 1 tablet PO PRN		

→ Close the MAR and return to Andrea Wang's chart. Click on **Nurses' Notes**. As you read the notes, consider the major concerns that emerge regarding this patient's care.

16. Create a list of concerns and a problem list based on the data you have collected thus far from the chart.

a. Concerns:

b. Problem list (nursing diagnoses and collaborative problems):

LESSON 28

Acute Spinal Cord Injury— Part II

📖 **Reading Assignment:** Nursing Management: Peripheral Nerve and Spinal Cord
Problems (Chapter 57)

Patient: Andrea Wang, Room 310

For this lesson, you will continue to care for Andrea Wang, a 20-year-old female admitted to the hospital following an acute spinal cord injury. You should have completed Lesson 27 prior to beginning this lesson.

💿 **CD-ROM Activity**

Go to the Supervisor's Office and sign in to work with Andrea Wang for the Tuesday 0700 shift. Proceed to the bulletin board in the Nurses' Station and find the location of the nursing report (Remember: you can also find this information by moving your cursor across the animated map in the upper right corner of your screen.)

1. Listen to report and record pertinent notes below.

2. Did anything in the report seem inconsistent? Is there anything else you wish the nurse would have addressed during report? Explain.

271

→ Go to Andrea Wang's room and click on **Vital Signs**.

3. Take a set of vital sign readings, including pain rating. Record these below and in the EPR.

Heart rate _____   Temperature _____

Respiratory rate _____   Oxygen saturation _____

Blood pressure _____   Pain rating/location _____

4. Based on Andrea Wang's vital signs, what nursing intervention is appropriate?

→ Next, click on **Physical**.

5. Collect all the physical examination data for Andrea Wang and record below and on the next page. Are any data out of the ordinary and/or unexpected?

Area Examined	Findings
Head and Neck	
Chest/Upper Extremities	

Area Examined **Findings**

Abdomen and
Lower Extremities

➤ Click on **Medications** and then on **Administer**. Observe the nurse give Andrea Wang her 0900 medications.

6. Which routine medication due at 0900 did the nurse fail to administer?

➤ Click on **Health History** and conduct a complete interview.

7. As you listen to the interview for each of the 12 health history categories, record significant data below and on the next page.

Area **Significant Data**

Perception/Self-Concept

Activity

Area	Significant Data
Sexuality/Reproduction	
Culture	
Nutrition-Metabolic	
Sleep-Rest	
Role/Relationship	

Area	Significant Data
Health Perception	
Elimination	
Cognitive/Perceptual	
Coping/Stress	
Value/Belief	

8. Now that you have collected data from the health history, the physical examination, and vital sign readings, revisit the problem list you developed in Lesson 27 (question 16b). Record that list in the left column below. Based on what you have learned, revise your list in the right column.

Original Problem List (from Lesson 27)	New Revised Problem List
Nursing diagnoses:	Nursing diagnoses:
Collaborative problems:	Collaborative problems:

➡ We will now make a virtual leap in time to Thursday. To do this, return to the Supervisor's Office and sign in again on the desktop computer. Click on **Reset** and select Andrea Wang for Thursday 1100. Next, find the location of the nursing report on Andrea Wang. Go to that location and listen to report.

9. Record significant data from report below.

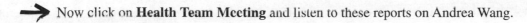 Now click on **Health Team Meeting** and listen to these reports on Andrea Wang.

10. Below, record the primary concerns of each of the health team members. When you have finished, go to the Nurses' Station and open Andrea Wang's chart. Click on **Health Team**, read each member's report, and add additional data below.

Case Manager

Social Worker

Clinical Nurse
Specialist

11. The clinical nurse specialist and other nurses mention the need to monitor Andrea Wang for autonomic dysreflexia. What is this? What are the symptoms? How is this condition managed?

➤ Click on **Nurses' Notes** and read the notes since Tuesday.

12. From the nurses' notes, what issues are evident regarding Andrea Wang's care?

13. You are asked to spend time with Andrea Wang going over measures to prevent skin break-down. Write down some ideas you have regarding what you should discuss with her. Refer to your textbook for ideas.

→ We will once again make a virtual leap in time and jump ahead to Friday. Return to the Supervisor's Office and sign in to work with Andrea Wang for the Friday shift. Proceed to the Nurses' Station and open her chart.

14. Read the nurses' notes from Thursday night. What complication developed?

15. What was the apparent cause of the complication?

16. Were Andrea Wang's symptoms consistent with those presented in the textbook? What were her symptoms?

Skeletal Fracture

──

 Reading Assignment: Nursing Assessment: Musculoskeletal System (Chapter 58)

Nursing Management: Musculoskeletal Problems (Chapter 59)

Patient: David Ruskin, Room 303

For this lesson, you are assigned to care for David Ruskin, a 31-year-old male patient who was hit by a car while riding his bike. This patient has, among many injuries, a fracture to his right arm.

CD-ROM Activity

Go to the Supervisor's Office and sign in to work with David Ruskin for Tuesday at 0700. Proceed to the Nurses' Station and open the patient's chart. Read the entire Physical & History, including the Emergency Department Report. (Remember to scroll down to read all pages.)

1. According to your textbook, the initial clinical manifestations of a fractured humerus can include the following: edema, bone deformity, decreased bone function, pain, ecchymosis, and crepitation. Describe the significance of those clinical findings below and on the next page. Then, compare these typical clinical findings with those described for David Ruskin in the Emergency Department Report. Circle those findings that are documented.

Clinical Finding	Significance
Edema	
Decreased function	

Clinical Finding	Significance
Pain	
Ecchymosis	
Crepitation	

2. What additional data were included in the Emergency Department Report regarding the fractured humerus?

 3. If you had done the initial ED assessment of the right arm, what additional data might you have included? *(Hint: Consult your textbook and review the "five Ps.")*

Now consider all the presenting injuries as documented in the Emergency Department Report. Consider how you would have prioritized your assessment if you had been working in the ER when David Ruskin was brought in.

4. Below, list all of David Ruskin's presenting injuries in the first column. In the second column, rank each injury according to what you believe to be the priority of assessment (highest = 1; next highest = 2, etc.) In the third column, indicate what impact these other injuries may have had on assessment of the fractured humerus (if any).

Presenting Injury	Priority of Assessment	Impact of Injury on Assessment of the Arm (if any)

 Click on **Diagnostics** in David Ruskin's chart. Read the x-ray report for Sunday at 1600.

5. Based on Dr. Kawasaki's report, circle the picture below that best represents the type of fracture David Ruskin has?

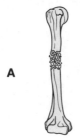

A

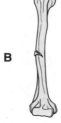

B

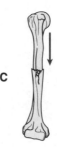

C

→ Now click on **Physicians' Orders** and review the orders for Sunday night through Tuesday morning. When you are finished, close the chart and access the patient's MAR (in the blue notebook on the counter.) Review David Ruskin's MAR.

6. Determine what routine medication(s) you will be giving to David Ruskin today during the day shift (0700–1500). Below, list the medication(s) you need to give, the reason why each is given, and the time each is due.

Medication	Why Given	Time Due

→ The night nurse is ready to start report on David Ruskin. Close the MAR, check the bulletin for location, and go to hear report.

7. Record significant data from report below.

8. What did you think about the report you were given? Were there any inconsistencies? Is there anything else you wish the nurse would have included in the report related to the fractured arm?

 9. Formulate a care plan for the day. Refer to Table 59-1 in your textbook and review the nursing care plan for a patient with a fracture. Below, list what you consider to be the top five priority nursing diagnoses and/or collaborative problem(s) from Table 59-1 that are applicable in this clinical situation (with the focus on the fractured humerus). In the second column, list some of the interventions you think would be appropriate for David Ruskin.

Nursing Diagnosis or Collaborative Problem	Intervention

➡ Go to David Ruskin's room and obtain a set of vital signs.

10. Record David Ruskin's vital signs below and then enter them in the EPR.

Heart rate _____   Temperature _____

Respiratory rate _____   Oxygen saturation _____

Blood pressure _____

➡ In David Ruskin's room, click on **Physical** and conduct a complete bedside examination.

11. Below, record your findings from David Ruskin's physical examination.

Area Examined	**Findings**
Head and Neck	
Chest/Upper Extremities	
Abdomen and Lower Extremities	

12. Consider all the data you have just collected. What interventions might you provide at this time? Is there anything missing? Is there anything that changes your plan of care?

➡ A nursing assistant tells you that David Ruskin seems to be in pain. Go to his room and assess the situation. First, obtain his pain rating. Then go to one of the computers that access the EPR and record his pain level there.

13. What medication(s) can be given to David Ruskin for the pain? What other data need to be assessed before you make a decision to give him a pain medication at this time?

Pain rating = _____

Medication(s) available:

Other symptoms:

Decision (choose one):

____ Medicate David Ruskin with _____

____ Do not medicate David Ruskin at this time.

Rationale:

→ It is time to give David Ruskin his 0900 medications. Go to his room and administer the medications.

Lunch time! Leave the floor and go to lunch.

→ After lunch, sign in again to work with David Ruskin for Tuesday 1100. Go to the Nurses' Station and access the patient's MAR. Note that David Ruskin has cefoxitin due at 1200. Before you give the medication, consider a few things about this drug. (You will probably want to refer to a drug handbook.)

14. What is the purpose of cefoxitin?

15. In what types of IV solution could you expect the cefoxitin to be diluted? (In other words, with what IV solutions is it compatible?)

16. How long should it take to administer 1 gram of cefoxitin?

→ Now access David Ruskin's EPR and find his CBC results.

17. What is David Ruskin's WBC count result?

18. What does this result mean?

➡ Check David Ruskin's body temperature trends over the last several days.

19. What do you see happening with his body temperature?

20. How are David Ruskin's WBC count and his temperature trends relevant in regard to giving him cefoxitin?

Osteomyelitis

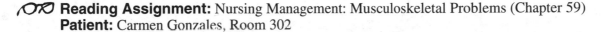 **Reading Assignment:** Nursing Management: Musculoskeletal Problems (Chapter 59)
Patient: Carmen Gonzales, Room 302

For this lesson, you are assigned to care for Carmen Gonzales, a 56-year-old female patient admitted to the hospital with type 2 diabetes mellitus, a leg infection, and osteomyelitis.

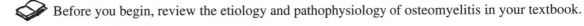 Before you begin, review the etiology and pathophysiology of osteomyelitis in your textbook.

1. What does the term *osteomyelitis* mean?

2. What is the difference between acute and chronic osteomyelitis?

   Acute osteomyelitis

   Chronic osteomyelitis

3. Osteomyelitis can occur by direct or indirect invasion. Describe the difference.

Direct invasion

Indirect invasion

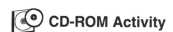 **CD-ROM Activity**

Go to the Supervisor's Office and sign in to work with Carmen Gonzales for the Tuesday 0700 shift. Proceed to the Nurses' Station and open her chart. Read the entire Physical & History, including the Emergency Department Record. (Scroll down to read all pages.)

4. The clinical manifestations of osteomyelitis can include both local and systemic symptoms. Common local and systemic signs and symptoms are listed below. Circle signs and symptoms consistent with Carmen Gonzales' history and physical examination findings on admission.

Local Symptoms	Systemic Symptoms
Severe bone pain	Fever
Swelling	Night sweats
Warmth at infection site	Chills
Restricted movement	Restlessness
	Nausea
	Malaise

5. Based on what you have read, identify the source of Carmen Gonzales' osteomyelitis and the type of invasion responsible for it.

**Type of Invasion
(circle one)**   **Source**

Direct   Indirect

➡ Now click on **Physicians' Orders** and read the orders for Sunday evening.

6. The following diagnostic tests are useful in the diagnosis and evaluation of osteomyelitis. Match each test with its corresponding description. Then circle Yes or No to indicate whether or not each diagnostic test was performed as part of Carmen Gonzales' admissions work-up.

	Diagnostic Test	**Description**
Yes No _____	MRI and CT scan	a. Initial test to determine causative organism.
Yes No _____	Wound culture	b. Helpful to identify boundaries of the infection.
Yes No _____	Blood leukocyte count	
Yes No _____	X-ray of affected extremity	c. Most definitive way to determine causative organism.
Yes No _____	Radionuclide bone scan	d. Elevated results of this test indicate infection.
Yes No _____	Bone/tissue biopsy	

e. Radiologic test that can identify osteomyelitis within 72 hours of onset.

f. Changes with this test do not appear until at least 10 days after onset of clinical symptoms.

➤ Click on **Diagnostics** and review the radiologic report for Sunday at 1600 hours. Compare this report with the pathophysiology of osteomyelitis as described in the textbook.

7. What finding is documented on the x-ray report that is consistent with osteomyelitis? What does this finding mean?

Finding documented on the x-ray report

Meaning

➤ Click on **Surgeons' Notes** and review the surgical report for Monday afternoon.

8. According to the textbook, collaborative care of osteomyelitis may include surgical debridement of the bony tissue. What type of surgery was performed in Carmen Gonzales' case? Did this include surgical debridement of the bone?

→ Now close the chart and go to the MAR in the blue notebook on the counter. Open Carmen Gonzales' MAR for today.

9. Determine what routine medication(s) (including the continuous IV) you will be giving to Carmen Gonzales today during the day shift (0700–1500). Below, list the medication(s) you need to give, the reason why each is given, and the time each is due.

Medication	Why Given	Time Due

→ You are aware that the cefoxitin has been ordered for Carmen Gonzales because of her leg infection. You decide to check the WBC done on Sunday night because you are curious (also, you are sure your nursing instructor will ask you about it). Close the MAR and go to the computer under the bookshelf to access the EPR. Find the hematology results for Carmen Gonzales.

10. Below, record Carmen Gonzales' hematology results for Sunday night. Explain what each result means.

Test	Result	What does this mean?
Hgb		
Hct		
WBC		

→ The night nurse is ready to give report on Carmen Gonzales. Close the EPR, check the bulletin board for report location, and go to hear the report.

11. Record significant data from the report below.

12. What did you think about the report you were given? Is there anything else you wish the nurse would have included in the report regarding osteomyelitis? If so, what?

→ It is now 0745. Go to Carmen Gonzales' room, click on **Vital Signs**, and obtain a full set of vital sign readings.

13. Record Carmen Gonzales' vital sign readings below and in the EPR.

Heart rate _____   Temperature _____

Respiratory rate _____   Oxygen saturation _____

Blood pressure _____   Pain rating _____

14. Based on what you have learned from obtaining Carmen Gonzales' vital signs, you should return to her room to give her what PRN medication? Why?

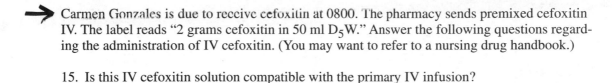 Carmen Gonzales is due to receive cefoxitin at 0800. The pharmacy sends premixed cefoxitin IV. The label reads "2 grams cefoxitin in 50 ml D$_5$W." Answer the following questions regarding the administration of IV cefoxitin. (You may want to refer to a nursing drug handbook.)

15. Is this IV cefoxitin solution compatible with the primary IV infusion?

16. Over what amount of time should you infuse this IV antibiotic?

17. If you are using an IV pump to deliver this medication piggyback, what rate (mL per hour) will you select to give this infusion?

   _____ mL/hour

➡ Now return to Carmen Gonzales' room and conduct a complete physical examination and health history.

18. After gathering data from the health history interview and physical examination, develop a plan of care for the day for Carmen Gonzales. Refer to Nursing Care Plan 59-3 in your textbook. Complete each of the nursing diagnoses on the next two paes by tailoring them to Carmen Gonzales' situation. Provide goals and interventions for each diagnosis. After the last diagnosis on p. 252, write another nursing diagnosis that seems appropriate based on what you know about this patient's case.

Nursing Diagnosis

Goal(s)

Interventions

Pain related to

as manifested by

Hyperthermia related to

as manifested by

Nursing Diagnosis	Goal(s)	Interventions
Impaired physical mobility related to _____ as manifested by _____		
Ineffective management of therapeutic regime related to _____ as manifested by _____		

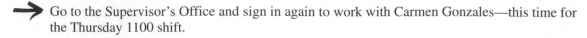 Go to the Supervisor's Office and sign in again to work with Carmen Gonzales—this time for the Thursday 1100 shift.

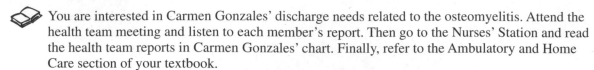 You are interested in Carmen Gonzales' discharge needs related to the osteomyelitis. Attend the health team meeting and listen to each member's report. Then go to the Nurses' Station and read the health team reports in Carmen Gonzales' chart. Finally, refer to the Ambulatory and Home Care section of your textbook.

19. Based on what you know and have read, what do you expect will be included in Carmen Gonzales' discharge instructions and follow-up care to manage her osteomyelitis?

Answers

Lesson 1 – The Continuum of Patient Care

1. d
2. c
3. a
4. b

5. Andrea Wang

6. Andrea Wang suffered an acute spinal cord injury. This is a very serious injury with the potential for multisystem involvement.

7. Sally Begay

8. Sally Begay has an acute problem that could potentially require aggressive medical intervention. She needs specific observation in the event her condition changes.

9. Ira Bradley

10. Ira Bradley has an acute exacerbation of a chronic illness. He is in the end stage of his disease; thus aggressive intensive care is not appropriate.

11. Transitional Care Settings: This stage of care is intermediary between acute and home care settings. Patients may need transitional care for a short period of time (days) or long period of time (months).

    Subacute Care: These settings provide postacute care for patients who no longer need acute care but are too sick to go to a nursing home or their own home. Typically, patients requiring subacute are chronically ill or have ongoing nursing care needs.

    Acute Rehabilitation Care: These settings also provide postacute level of care, but acute rehabilitation units typically specialize in therapy for patients with neurologic or physical injuries (head injury, spinal cord injury, cerebral vascular accident, etc). These settings usually have multiple disciplines such as physical therapy, occupational therapy, and speech therapy involved in patient care.

    Long-Term Care: This term refers to the care of patients with functional self-care deficits. Often individuals requiring long-term care have severe developmental disabilities, mental impairments, or physical deficits requiring continuous medical or nursing management. Persons in these settings are usually referred to as *residents* as opposed to *patients* or *clients*. These settings include skilled nursing facilities and nursing homes.

Home Health Care: This is a broad term used to describe care delivered in the home setting. This care may be provided intermittently or on a full-time, 24-hour-a-day basis. The number of visits may vary from a single visit to multiple visits over a period of years. The type of care delivered varies considerably and can include education, health maintenance, and specific treatments.

Hospice Care: This is care provided to individuals who are terminally ill and who choose to die in the comfort of their own home. Hospice provides care for persons in the last phases of incurable disease so that they may live as fully and comfortably as possible.

12. Home care

13. Sally Begay has several risk factors for recurrent pulmonary infection. She also has strong family history, placing her at risk for several problems. Her primary need for home care at this point is education; however it must be culturally sensitive to her traditional Navajo lifestyle.

14. Home care or hospice care

15. Two answers are possibly correct for Ira Bradley. He has several problems that could potentially benefit from home health visits. He has nutritional issues, medication regime issues, and family issues. It is possible that this patient could benefit from hospice care at some point in the near future as well. He is terminally ill and reaching the end stage of his illness. Hospice care is something that should be explored as a possibility at some point.

16. Acute rehabilitation care

17. Andrea Wang has an acute spinal cord injury and will need a great deal of physical rehabilitation. In addition, the rehabilitation care will address many of the social issues that she and her family seem to be facing.

18. The textbook chapter describes case management as a central focus of community-based and home health care. The focus of case management is on the coordination of patient care during the entire episode of illness across all settings. Case management strives to provide quality care along a continuum. The continuum of patient care means that different settings accommodate the needs of the patient—from acute hospitalization admission to rehabilitation and home care.

19. Focus of the Nurse Case Manager: The nurse case manager looks at the whole picture, identifies a variety of problems from the patient's perspective, and attempts to coordinate the care considering the role of all care givers in all settings.

Focus of the Clinical Nurse Specialist: The clinical nurse specialist tends to focus on nursing management and treatment, such as medication regime, nutrition, hydration, ADL, etc. This person may make specific recommendations regarding the management of a specific care issue.

Focus of the Social Worker: The focus of the social worker tends to be on family issues, support systems, and financial considerations, to name a few. The social worker explores options and solutions for issues related to these concerns.

Lesson 2 – Adult Development

1. Young Adulthood: Focus is on gaining independence from parents, establishing self-concept and self-identity; development of close personal relationships; marriage and starting a family; raising young children. Focus may also be on obtaining education, finding a job, or starting a career.

   Middle Adulthood: Focus is on raising children or adjusting to grown children and possibly the role of grandparent; adjusting to aging parents; continuing a productive life. Realization of the finiteness of life is common; many experience an increased spiritual focus.

   Older Adulthood: Adjustments to changes in health, income, and social relationships occur. Restructuring of family roles and responsibilities occurs with retirement. Living arrangements may change if there is a decline in physical capability to meet daily living needs. Loss of spouse is another characteristic common in this stage.

2. Carmen Gonzales, 56, middle adulthood
   Sally Begay, 58, middle adulthood
   Ira Bradley, 43, middle adulthood
   David Ruskin, 31, early to middle adulthood
   Andrea Wang, 20, young adulthood

3. All choices are factors that play a role in adult development: age, activity level, culture, independence, general health, family interactions, living arrangement, self-concept, and self-esteem

4. Andrea Wang

   Consistent Tasks. Before the injury, she was very typical in most areas. Friends were important; she had developed a close relationship with her boyfriend; she had many outside interests. She was going to college, had career goals, was independent from her parents, and made her own choices.

   Inconsistent Tasks or Concerns: Spinal cord injury has placed her in a dependent role. Future is uncertain; fearful of the impact of her injury on all aspects of her life—friends, boyfriend, role with parents, ability to complete school, etc. This injury will no doubt interfere, at least initially, with developmental tasks of young adulthood.

5. David Ruskin

   Consistent Tasks: David Ruskin is very consistent with a typical 31-year-old in almost all ways. He is married and has a close relationship with his wife; they are expecting a baby. He is independent from his parents and has established himself in the adult world. He has many friends, providing a strong social support network. He is motivated to maintain health though nutrition and exercise. He is in school and is interested in being in control of his care. He is confident he can manage his care with some help from his wife and friends.

   Inconsistent Tasks or Concerns: There are really no areas of inconsistency with tasks or concerns regarding this patient being able to meet tasks. He is agreeable to needing help temporarily but sees this as only an inconvenience.

6. Answers will vary widely. Important key concepts include focus on maintaining and gaining independence; identification of realistic goals; identification of motivators for health care. Both patients consider themselves young and healthy; both of them dislike the dependent role. Both patients value education and are motivated. David Ruskin is well established in his role of independent man with family; Andrea Wang is in early task development of independence from family.

Lesson 3 – Health History and Physical Examination—Part I

1. The primary purpose is the collection of data—this is the assessment phase of the nursing process. The data are used to identify patient problems, set goals, and carry out interventions.

2. The medical history is a standard format designed to collect data to be used primarily by the physician to diagnose a health problem; it is usually based on a body systems format. The nursing history is geared to collection of data to identify patient problems (nursing diagnoses) and treatment of these problems through nursing intervention.

3. Subjective data consist of what the patient tells you. A great deal of subjective data is gained from conducting the history. Objective data are observed findings. Most objective data is gained during the process of examination.

4. Ordinarily, the best source of subjective data is the patient. However, the reliability or ability of a patient to provide a history may be an issue. Other sources for the history include the patient's family, significant others, and sometimes the chart.

5. j
6. h
7. g
8. k
9. f
10. a
11. d
12. i
13. a
14. b
15. f
16. a
17. j
18. c
19. h
20. d
21. e
22. b
23. k
24. f
25. i
26. a
27. b
28. k

29. History of present illness: Questions concerning why the patient came here; the onset and description of the patient's current problem

    Family history: Information regarding blood relatives and diseases with familial tendencies

    Social history: Occupation, alcohol intake, smoking, etc.

    Medical history: Past medical problems—past surgeries, admissions, etc.

    Current medications: List of medications patient is currently taking, including dose and length of time taking the medication

    Review of systems: A review of questions structured in a framework by body systems.

30. The Physical & History provides valuable information to enhance the nurse's understanding of the patient's condition. The nurse should review this data so that baseline data can be identified. The nurse should also recognize data that are abnormal.

31. Data that are out of ordinary:

    Patient has risk factors for diabetes, hypertension, CVA, and coronary artery disease.

    Patient has coronary artery disease; had an MI 5 years ago; has angina and mild CHF; has hypertension and COPD; is taking medications to manage hypertension and angina

    Patient has productive cough, chest pain with coughing, fatigue, and dyspnea; has orthopnea; no edema.

    Decreased appetite; some nausea and vomiting.

32. Health Perception/Health Promotion: Usually views self as "healthy." States she "coughs a lot" and that it hurts more this past year. Sees doctor and medicine man to gain information to care for herself.

    Nutritional/Metabolic: Has own teeth; no problems; no dentures or bridges. States she eats "just about anything." Food preferences include cheese. Eats fruits and vegetables "once in a while." Does not like sweets and desserts. Milk intolerance—makes her feel bloated and gives her diarrhea. Weight described as stable over past couple years; thinks she may have lost a little weight during last month.

    Elimination: Normally has one BM per day; however, has not had a BM in 2 days while at hospital. No problems with urinary elimination, no changes in pattern

    Activity/Exercise: Presently, patient verbalizes fatigue and easily becomes short of breath. At home she works with farm animals, describes getting "lots of exercise." Recreation includes playing with grandchildren and visiting family. She thinks she will be able to care for herself when she goes home. She believes the shortness of breath may slow her down. Son and wife are available to help.

    Sleep/Rest: Difficulty sleeping in hospital. At home, sleep is usually restful; however, during the last week she has had sleeping difficulty due to shortness of breath—needs pillows to sleep. Needs to rest frequently. Sleep rituals include reading a book and watching TV.

    Cognitive/Perceptual: No problems with language. Speaks English, Navajo, and Dinebizaad Navajo. No problems with memory recall; no problems or changes in vision or hearing; no headaches. Likes to learn by having someone show her things.

    Self-Perception/Self-Concept: Describes herself by her Indian tribe. She states, "I live on my mother's land." Effect of illness has caused her to be very concerned about things at home. Is worried about whether the animals are cared for.

    Role-Relationship: Married. Describes relationship with husband as close. Has two children. Works at home on their farm raising animals—worries that her illness will interfere with this activity because husband cannot do this all himself. Son and his wife are available to help out.

    Sexuality/Reproductive: Patient is menopausal; has two children.

Coping/Stress Tolerance: <u>Biggest stress at this time is concern over the farm and her husband managing things alone</u>. Family usually able to work problems out by talking things over. Support systems include friends and neighbors, many of whom are described as "clan relatives." Patient states, "We all work together."

Value/Belief: She values both the hospital and the medicine man. Most important things to her are family, animals, friends, and her people.

33. See answer 32 for underlining of data that are out of ordinary, indicating negative function.

34. Answers to this question will vary. The nurse on the CD failed to ask many important questions. Some key areas that should be addressed include questions related to the impact of illness on the activity level, risk factors for other health problems, educational needs, etc.

Lesson 4 – Health History and Physical Examination—Part II

1. Focused examination: A focused examination is usually a short examination that addresses a chief complaint and all body systems that might be affected.

   Comprehensive examination: This is a detailed examination focusing on all body systems, regardless of whether there is a chief compliant or not.

   Bedside or shift-to-shift examination: This is an abbreviated examination looking at all the primary body systems, but not in depth. The purpose of this type of examination is to identify baseline data and then to monitor for changes from baseline each shift.

2. Inspection: This is what you see—a visual examination of the entire person (general inspection) or a specific body area or body part.

   Palpation: This is what you feel—palpation includes touching to determine texture, tenderness, warmth, pulsation, masses, organ enlargement, etc.

   Percussion: This is a technique in which the examiner elicits sounds from underlying structures—an indirect technique. Occasionally, the examiner will conduct direct percussion to determine tenderness (over sinuses or kidney).

   Auscultation: This technique involves use of a stethoscope to listen to sounds produced by the body. Typical sounds to auscultate include heart sounds, lung sounds, bowel sounds, and blood pressure. Vascular sounds (bruits) may also be auscultated.

3. HEENT: Examination of the head and neck—includes eyes, ears, nose, mouth, and throat.

   Cardiopulmonary: Includes examination of the thorax for heart and lung assessment. Peripheral vascular assessment includes adequacy of perfusion (i.e., pulse checks, capillary refill, warmth, edema).

   Neurologic: May include mental status cranial nerve assessment, cerebellar assessment, and nervous system findings.

   Musculoskeletal: Examination of the major muscle groups for symmetry, strength, and range of motion.

   Gastrointestinal: Examination of the abdomen, including inspection, auscultation, and palpation.

   Genitourinary: Examination of the urinary tract and genitalia. This was deferred.

4. RR = 24/minute
   O_2 sat = 87% on RA
   Tactile fremitis greater on right side
   Crackles auscultated in right middle and lower lobes of lung

5. Keep in mind that modesty is an important concern among the Navajo; you will want to take measure to limit exposure. Ask permission before you touch the patient. Navajo typically are quiet individuals and may not elaborate in conversation unless encouraged to do so.

6. **Head and Neck**
   Techniques used:
   Observed six cardinal fields of gaze.
   Observed facial movements (CN VII).
   Observed tongue movement (CN XII).
   Inspected oral mucosa.
   Observed range of motion of neck.
   Palpated lymph nodes.
   Inspected for jugular distention.
   Palpated carotid pulses.
   Mistakes:
   The nurse documented PERRLA, but this was never performed.

   Chest/Upper Extremities
   Techniques used:
   Auscultated lungs (anterior and posterior).
   Auscultated for heart sounds.
   Palpated for thoracic excursion.
   Palpated radial pulses.
   Palpated capillary refill.
   Checked grasp strength of hands.
   Mistakes:
   Should do chest inspection, but did not do this.
   Correct technique to palpate symmetric thoracic expansion includes standing behind patient, placing thumbs on T-12, and asking patient to take a deep breath. Then watch movement of thumbs—should be symmetric.

   Abdomen and Lower Extremities
   Techniques used:
   Inspected abdomen.
   Auscultated abdomen.
   Palpated abdomen.
   Palpated posterior tibial pulses.
   Palpated pedal pulses.
   Palpated capillary refill.
   Palpated and inspected for edema.
   Mistakes:
   Inspected abdomen without lifting gown. Inspection of abdomen should include movements, surface characteristics, and shape. This cannot be done through a gown. Also, palpated the posterior tibial pulse, but did not document the findings.

   Vital Signs
   Findings:
   Temperature: 99.6° F
   Oxygen saturation: 93% on 1L/NC
   Pulse: 96
   Blood pressure: 150/76
   Respiratory rate: 20
   Pain rating: 5–6

Head and Neck
Findings:
Has intact oculomotor function and facial symmetry.
<u>Oral mucosa is dry.</u>
No enlargement of lymph nodes.
No JVD.
Carotid pulses are bilaterally equal with +3 amplitude.

Chest/Upper Extremities
Findings:
<u>Crackles auscultated in right middle and lower lobes both anteriorly and posteriorly.</u>
  Other areas clear.
S_1 and S_2 heart sounds auscultated; no abnormal sounds noted.
Excursion normal.
Chest expansion bilaterally symmetric.
Radial pulses equal bilaterally with +3 amplitude.
Capillary refill is <3 seconds.
Grip is strong and equal bilaterally.

Abdomen and Lower Extremities
Findings:
Abdomen appears symmetric on inspection.
Bowel sounds auscultated × 4.
Abdomen is soft, nontender; no masses palpated.
Dorsalis pedis pulses palpated +2 left foot, +3 right foot.
Capillary refill is <3 seconds bilaterally.
No edema.

7. See findings underlined in answer 6.

8. The nurse should make a patient problem list and use the data to identify nursing diagnoses and collaborative problems on which to base a plan of care.

Lesson 5 – Patient Teaching

1. Compliance Approach: Nurse independently develops, implements, and evaluates a teaching plan. The patient is a passive recipient of the teaching experience.

   Empowerment Approach: Patient and family identify goals—this approach is particularly effective when caring for a patient with a chronic condition. Nurse assists patient in development of plan to attain his or her individual goals. Optimizes patient knowledge and autonomy.

2. Although a number of data entries are acceptable, the following are particularly significant:
   Has osteomyelitis.
   Is diabetic.
   Patient's preference for speaking Spanish poses a language barrier—will require a translator.
   Does not understand why she has foot infections.
   Likes demonstration for instruction.
   Feels comfortable with family traditions.

3. Although a number of data entries are acceptable, the following are particularly significant:

   Multiple diagnoses—osteomyelitis, type 2 DM, CHF, CAD.

   Previous admission 5 months ago for infection of right foot.

   Patient education regarding type 2 diabetes mellitus provided during previous admission.

   Upon this admission, patient reported she takes medications for her heart and diabetes, but she was unable to recall the drug names.

   Patient in a lot of pain; having trouble caring for herself.

   She is Hispanic; Spanish is preferred language.

   Works 4 hours a day; husband retired; living on fixed income.

4. **Description from textbook:**

   Age: Age is defined primarily in terms of developmental stage—for example, young adults and older adults may be receptive to different things.

   Culture: Nurse must keep in mind culturally sensitive care. Patients should be asked to share their beliefs about illness and health so that the nurse will have an understanding of their values. Plan should be congruent with these values.

   Educational Level: Need to assess reading and cognitive ability because these variables can affect the ability of the patient to comprehend what is being taught.

   Self-Efficacy: This is a person's belief in his or her ability to understand and follow a regime or recommendation.

   Psychologic State: Factors that can negatively affect patient motivation and readiness to learn include anxiety and stress.

   Application to Carmen Gonzales:

   Age: Age is 56; refers to herself as "old now" on several occasions.

   Culture: Hispanic; considers herself "American"; preferred language is Spanish.

   Educational Level: No information available.

   Self-Efficacy: Statements indicate a feeling of hopelessness and a need for someone to take care of her; statements reveal that she is not sure whether she can ever walk again.

   Psychologic State: Patient has a somewhat flat affect, has pain in her leg, and seems anxious about her condition. She voices fears about her ability to get better.

5. Used a translator.

   Was very respectful.

   Used a very calming voice.

   Did not rush—patient has a slow pace; nurse kept pace with her.

   Allowed pauses, let her answer.

   Asked her permission.

6. Table 5-1 Assessment of Characteristics That Affect Patient Teaching

Characteristic	Key Questions
Readiness to learn	O What has your physician or nurse practitioner told you about your health problem?
	O What behaviors could make your problem better or worse?
Biophysical	X What is the primary diagnosis?
	X Are there additional diagnoses?
	X Is the patient acutely ill?
	X How old is the patient?
	O What is the patient's current mental status?
	X What is the patient's hearing ability? Visual ability? Motor ability?
	X Is the patient fatigued? In pain?
	X What medications is the patient on? How might these affect learning?
Psychologic	O Does the patient appear anxious? Afraid? Depressed? Defensive?
	O Is the patient in a state of denial?
Sociocultural	X Does the patient have family or close friends?
	O What is the patient's belief regarding his or her illness or treatment?
	O Is the proposed change consistent with the patient's cultural values?
Socioeconomic	X Does the patient work?
	X What is the patient's occupation?
	X What is the patient's living arrangement?
Learning style	O Does the patient "learn best" through visual (reading), auditory (tape or lecture), or physical stimuli (demonstration)?
	O In what kind of environment does the patient learn best? Formal classroom? Informal setting, such as home or office? Alone or among peers? What prior learning experiences were helpful?

7. Rose Simpson, Case Manager
   Concerns:
   - Coordination of care—has multiple system problems, must be sure to manage all of these effectively.
   - Patient education—need to manage blood glucose levels, reduce lower extremity infections, lower risk for development of recurrent heart failure.
   - Family support for care may be limited; home care may be necessary.
   - Follow-up care.

   Louise Johnson, CNS
   Goals:
   - Manage her blood glucose.
   - Reduce incidence of infection.
   - Concern for her cardiac status; follow up with cardiologist for cardiac work-up.

   Kris Holmes, MSW
   4 main areas of concern:
   - Finances.
   - Help from children may be an issue.
   - Decreasing social network.
   - Support networks for access to education, transportation, etc.

8. Lists may vary significantly, but here are several of the most important teaching issues:
   Dietary management
   Wound care
   Medications
   Activity
   How to reduce risk of infection

Specific disease education:
    Congestive heart failure
    Hypertension
    Diabetes mellitus, type 2
    Social networks/agencies to provide services

9. Communication: Nurse should indicate the use of a translator. If written materials are being used, assessment of reading level is important, as well as finding materials written in Spanish.

Method of teaching: Patient indicated she learns best by watching—if possible, this should be a component of the learning, perhaps by using videos.

Involvement of patient and family: Since this is chronic illness, the nurse should use the empowerment approach, thus setting goals with Carmen Gonzales and her family. This is likely to increase compliance.

Lesson 6 – Stress Response

1. c
2. a
3. b

4. Bike accident/multiple trauma
Fracture to right humerus
Closed head injury
Lacerations and bruising to head
Road rash to right flank and right lateral calf
Surgical procedure (ORIF) to fix arm
Pain

5. c
6. a
7. a, b
8. a
9. b
10. b
11. a
12. a
13. b
14. a

15. ↑ Blood pressure
↓ Gastrointestinal motility
↑ Heart rate
↑ Perspiration
↑ Respiratory rate
Pupils—Dilation

16. Temperature: 99.1° F
Pulse: 83
Respiration: 20
Blood pressure: 145/70

17. Stage of Resistance

18. **Current Possible Sources of Stress:**
   Post-op recovery.
   "Feels stupid."
   Wants to get back on bike.
   Has pain.
   Limitation in mobility and self-care activities.
   Wife is pregnant.
   Not sleeping well in the hospital.
   Has headaches.
   Marriage; interracial couple.
   Is "out of action."
   Worried about keeping up at work.

   Factors That Help to Resist Stress:
   Sleeps well at home.
   Has lots of energy.
   Very interested in proper nutrition.
   Maintains stable/ideal weight.
   Does not smoke/does not use drugs.
   Moderate alcohol use (1 to 3 glasses of wine a week).
   Excellent shape—well-conditioned athlete.

19. The following coping resources apply: robust health, communication skills, self-efficacy, high energy level, collection of information, high morale, social networks, adequate finances

20. The main stressors seem to be pain, regaining independence, and concern for keeping up with work. Nursing measures that will benefit him the most include pain management, providing him with educational materials to read to help him feel and/or gain more control over his recovery, and helping him consider how his social and family networks can help him best during time of recovery.

21. David Ruskin is managing his stress very well. Since his injury is not a threat to life or limb, he seems to be approaching his recovery very pragmatically, and there are no major concerns at this time. None of the diagnoses listed in Table 7-9 are applicable to David Ruskin; however an argument could be made that some of these are "risk for" diagnoses.

Lesson 7 – Complementary and Alternative Therapies

1. F
2. T
3. F
4. F
5. T

6. Complementary therapies are used in addition to conventional treatments prescribed by the health care provider. Alternative therapies may include the same interventions as complementary therapy; however, these are frequently the *primary* treatment modality replacing conventional Western medical care.

7. e
8. d
9. h
10. l
11. i
12. b
13. k

14. g
15. a
16. j
17. f
18. c

19. **Carmen Gonzales**

Complementary therapies most likely to be accepted and/or helpful:
Latin-American practices: May be accepting of some traditional folk remedies consistent with Latin-American practices; would need to explore this.
Relaxation: May be very helpful in reducing anxiety.
Guided imagery: Since she is in a lot of pain, this may help to manage pain.
Therapeutic touch: May be very helpful to manage pain and anxiety.
Massage therapy: May be very helpful to produce needed relaxation.
Herbal therapy: May be very accepting since herbs are commonly used as part of Latino folk remedies.

Complementary therapies less likely to be accepted and/or helpful:
Chiropractic therapy: No real indication for this.
Native-American practices: Patient not Native-American; may not be accepting of this.
Traditional Chinese: Probably would not value this.
Hypnotherapy: May or may not be helpful.
Acupuncture: May or may not be helpful.
Biofeedback: Probably too anxious to do well with this.

David Ruskin

Complementary therapies most likely to be accepted and/or helpful:
Relaxation: Since he describes himself as spiritual, this may be very effective.
Guided imagery: May be very effective to manage pain.
Therapeutic touch: May or may not be effective.
Massage therapy: May be effective for relieving stress.
Herbal therapy: He may be open to this since he is very interested in nutrition.

Complementary therapies less likely to be accepted and/or helpful:
Chiropractic therapy: Not indicated for fractures.
Native-American practices: Probably would have little interest in this.
Latin-American practices: Probably would have little interest in this.
Traditional Chinese practices: Probably would have little interest in this.
Hypnotherapy: May or may not be effective.
Acupuncture: Probably not indicated for his acute pain.
Biofeedback: May be effective, but he has acute injuries.

Sally Begay

Complementary therapies most likely to be accepted and/or helpful:
Native-American practices: Has specifically indicated interest; values this type of therapy.
Relaxation: May be effective; many Native-American individuals are interested.
Herbal therapy: She may have interest in this since it may be consistent with some Native-American practices.

Complementary therapies less likely to be accepted and/or helpful:
Chiropractic therapy: Probably not indicated for her condition.
Latin-American practices: Probably would have little interest in this.
Traditional Chinese practices: Probably would have little interest in this.
Hypnotherapy: May or may not be effective.

Guided imagery: Not having pain; probably not indicated.
Acupuncture: Probably not indicated.
Therapeutic touch: May or may not be effective—may depend on the practitioner.
Biofeedback: May or may not be effective.
Massage therapy: May or may not be effective for relieving stress.

Ira Bradley

Complementary therapies most likely to be accepted and/or helpful:
Relaxation: May be effective to help manage stress.
Guided imagery: May be very effective to manage chronic pain.
Therapeutic touch: May be very effective in relief of pain and stressors.
Herbal therapy: He may have interest in this to help reduce nausea, pain, depression, and discomforts. May be open to it, especially if he is not satisfied with medication therapy or in the hope that anything may help improve how he feels.

Complementary therapies less likely to be accepted and/or helpful:
Chiropractic therapy: Probably not indicated for his condition.
Native-American practices: Probably would have little interest in this.
Latin-American practices: Probably would have little interest in this.
Traditional Chinese practices: Probably would have little interest in this.
Hypnotherapy: May or may not be effective.
Acupuncture: Probably not indicated.
Biofeedback: May or may not be effective.
Massage therapy: May or may not be effective for relieving stress.

Andrea Wang

Complementary therapies most likely to be accepted and/or helpful:
Traditional Chinese practices: Should explore this—may be something she is familiar with. She and her parents may see significant value in this therapy.
Relaxation: May be effective to help manage stress.
Guided imagery: May be very effective to manage stress.
Therapeutic touch: May be very effective in relief of stress.
Massage therapy: May be effective for relieving stress.
Herbal therapy: She may have interest in this part of traditional Chinese therapy

Complementary therapies less likely to be accepted and/or helpful:
Chiropractic therapy: Not indicated for acute spinal cord injury.
Native-American practices: Probably would have little interest in this.
Latin-American practices: Probably would have little interest in this.
Hypnotherapy: May or may not be effective.
Acupuncture: Probably not indicated for paralysis, but you might explore this.
Biofeedback: May or may not be effective.

20. There are really no right or wrong answers here. Answers can be highly individualized.

Lesson 8 – Pain

Pain Assessment Tool—David Ruskin
Tuesday 0800

Etiology (disease process and physical findings associated with pain) _____

Fracture to right arm, chest contusion, closed head injury

Type of Pain (circle one) ⟶ (acute)   chronic nonmalignant   malignant

Location of Pain (indicate location of pain using figure in box)

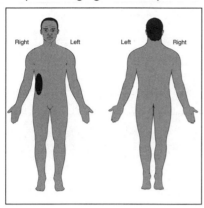

Description of the Pain Pattern

Pain in chest—especially when he takes a deep breath

Pain Intensity

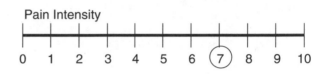

0   1   2   3   4   5   6   (7)   8   9   10

Description of the Pain Quality

Sharp pain in chest

Variables Affecting the Pain Experience

Affective   *Very calm*

Behavioral

Cognitive   *Has closed head injury—could affect*

Record of Pain Medications Given and Effectiveness

Day	Medication, Dose, and Time Given	Effectiveness
Sunday	*Fentanyl 1 mg IV 1615*	*Unknown*
Monday	*Ketorolac 30 mg IV 2330* *0600* *Oxycodone 5-10 mg PO* *@ 2400, 0400, 0800, 1030, 1500, 2100*	*Unknown*
Tuesday	*Oxycodone 5 mg* *0400*	*Unknown*

Pain Assessment Tool—Ira Bradley
Tuesday 0800

Etiology (disease process and physical findings associated with pain) _Candidiasis in mouth_

_____ _late-stage HIV, pneumonia, Kaposi's sarcoma_ _____

Type of Pain (circle one) ⟶ acute   chronic nonmalignant   (malignant)

Location of Pain (indicate location of pain using figure in box)

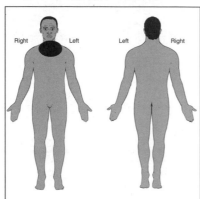

Right   Left   Left   Right

Description of the Pain Pattern

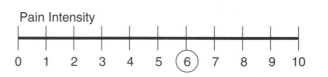

Chest and throat

Pain Intensity

0 1 2 3 4 5 (6) 7 8 9 10

Description of the Pain Quality

Dull, achy in chest—
"Burning"

Variables Affecting the Pain Experience

Affective   _Depressed_

Behavioral   _Family problems. Knows he is not_
getting better.

Cognitive   _Alert_

Record of Pain Medications Given and Effectiveness

Day	Medication, Dose, and Time Given	Effectiveness
Sunday	_None_	_Unknown_
Monday	_Oxycodone 10 mg PO_ _@ 0800_	_Unknown_
Tuesday	_Oxycodone 10 mg PO_ _@ 0400_	_Unknown_

2. The nursing documentation regarding the effectiveness of pain medication would have been helpful. Both patients should be asked about the quality of their pain.

3. **Similarities:**
   Both have similar pain rating (6 and 7).
   Both have same pain medication prescribed for moderate pain.

   Differences:
   David Ruskin has acute pain; Ira Bradley has chronic pain from malignant condition.
   The variables surrounding the pain experiences are very different.
   David Ruskin is receiving more pain medication than Ira Bradley.
   David Ruskin expects to get better; Ira Bradley does not expect this.

4. 1 to 3: mild pain
   4 to 6: moderate pain
   7 to 10: severe pain

5. David Ruskin is experiencing severe pain.
   Ira Bradley is experiencing moderate pain.

6. David Ruskin received pain medication. Ideally, both patients should have been offered pain medication. Pain ratings over 3 (moderate to severe pain) should be treated—according to the patient's needs. At the very least, the nurse should have offered a pain medication. It is possible Ira Bradley was asked and did not want pain medications. It is also possible that the nurse does not acknowledge his pain (it may not seem like he is in pain). However, this is never a valid reason to forgo medicating a patient for pain.

7. Step 1—Mild; Nonopioids (ASA, acetaminophen, NSAIDs)
   Step 2—Mild to moderate; Continue step 1 agents and add adjuvant drugs (codeine, oxycodone).
   Step 3—Moderate to severe; Replace step 2 agents with step 3 agents (morphine, hydromorphone).

8. Tylenol was ordered only for fever. You should recommend that this order be changed so that it could be given for mild pain as well. Otherwise, orders seem appropriate.

9. David Ruskin might benefit from positioning, cold therapy, distraction, imagery, and relaxation.
   Ira Bradley might benefit from positioning, distraction, imagery, and relaxation.

10. a
11. d
12. c
13. a
14. d

Lesson 9 – Inflammation and Infection

1. The bacteria cause destruction of the cell membrane or cell nucleus and produce lethal toxins.

2. a. Type 2 diabetes mellitus
   b. CHF
   c. CAD

3. Pain and swelling to the foot; fever and nausea × 2 days; vomiting × 24 hours; severe headache, fatigue, and shortness of breath.

4. Temperature 101.1° F
   Heart rate 95
   Respiratory rate 22
   Blood pressure 145/80

5. Fever: Caused by endogenous pyrogenic cytokines—indicates systemic response to inflammation/infection.

   Increased heart rate and respiratory rate: Caused from increased metabolic rate associated with fever.

   Malaise, nausea, and anorexia: Associated with systemic inflammation; cause not well understood, but probably has to do with activation of WBCs.

   Pain in the leg: Localized pain is associated with inflammation to the tissue.

6. Necrosis refers to death of tissue within a given area.

7. Gangrenous necrosis is often caused by ischemic injury—i.e., impaired circulation to the lower legs. Diabetes is commonly associated with poor perfusion of tissue to the lower extremities.

8. Although the physician documented evidence of an infectious process with the physical examination, the CBC helps the physician understand the process of the infection. The wound culture helps the physician determine what organism is causing the infection. This is especially helpful when ordering antibiotics.

9. This is a surgical procedure to remove necrotic tissue. Before the wound can heal, it must be "converted" to a clean wound. This is part of the collaborative care for wound healing.

10. Dressing change q8h.

11. This order does not indicate the type of dressing change that should be done (dry dressing or packed dressing), nor does it specify types of materials.

12. Hgb 11.4 (low)   Neutrophil segs 70%
    Hct 33.6 (low)   Neutrophil bands 2%
    RBC 4.2   Lymphocytes 14% (low)
    Platelets 496 (high)   Monocytes 9% (high)
    WBC 18.2 (high)   Eosinophils 4%
                                      Basophils 1%

    The hemoglobin and hematocrit are both low, which may be associated with anemia. Platelets are slightly elevated (normal 150–400), which may be associated with acute infection. The WBC is significantly elevated, indicating inflammation and infection. The WBC differential counts are close to normal; monocytes are slightly high; lymphocytes are low. This is the most surprising result because if the infection is acute, we expect bands to be elevated; if the infection is chronic, we expect lymphocytes and monocytes to be elevated.

13. Cefoxitin 2 grams IVPG q 6 hours.
    Times the medication is due on Tuesday: 0300, 0900, 1500, 2100

14. Acetaminophen 650 mg PO: PRN order for fever or for pain—both can be associated with the inflammation.

    Morphine 2–5 mg IM: PRN order for severe pain; can be given every 1–2 hours.

    Oxycodone 10 mg PO: PRN order for moderate pain; can be given every 4 hours.

15. Classification: Second-generation cephalosporin antibiotic

    Action: Bactericidal action—binds to bacterial cell wall membrane. Is considered a broad-spectrum drug, active against many gram-positive and gram-negative organisms.

    Indications: Primarily used for respiratory, skin, bone, and joint infections, as well as urinary tract and gynecologic infections.

    Contradictions/Precautions: Do not use in patients who are hypersensitive to other cephalosporins or who have had allergic reaction to penicillin. Use cautiously in patients with renal impairment.

    Major Adverse Effects: Pseudomembranous colitis, anaphylaxis, superinfection.

    Typical Dose: 1–2 grams q 4–6 hours IM or IV.

    IV Administration: Give as intermittent IV infusion over 15 to 30 minutes.

16. Elevation of extremity: Elevation helps to reduce the edema and increase venous return.

    Prevention of infection: Since Carmen Gonzales has a "clean wound" in the post-op period, nurse must carry out measures to prevent infection in the wound.

    Monitor vital signs: Changes in vital signs may be indicative of changes in the wound healing process.

    Monitor/encourage adequate nutritional and fluid intake: Fluid replacement is needed because of increased losses from fever and exudate formation. Adequate protein, carbohydrate, and fat intake is necessary to promote wound healing.

17. b
18. b
19. d
20. a
21. c

Lesson 10 – HIV—Part I

1. He has been unable to eat, drink, or take his medications the last couple of days. He has become short of breath, very weak, and disoriented. He fell at home and hit his head, causing a laceration.

2. HIV phase: AIDS
   Rationale: Ira Bradley meets several of the CDC criteria:
                 Fungal infections
                 Pneumocystis carinii pneumonia
                 Kaposi's sarcoma
                 Wasting syndrome

3. **Clinical Findings**

Pneumocystis carinii pneumonia

Typical Findings According to Textbook: Nonproductive cough, hypoxemia, shortness of breath, fatigue, night sweats.

Ira Bradley's Findings: According to history and clinical findings, he had all these except for night sweats. He has oxygen saturation of only 85% on admission.

Kaposi's sarcoma

Typical Findings According to Textbook: Firm and flat, raised or nodular, hyper-pigmented, multicentric lesions.

Ira Bradley's Findings: Unknown. Chart indicates only that he has Kaposi's sarcoma on thigh.

Candida (oral candidiasis)

Typical Findings According to Textbook: Whitish-yellow patches in mouth, esophagus, and GI tract.

Ira Bradley's Findings: Chart does not describe the lesions—only says they are present in his mouth and throat.

Diagnostic Tests

Pneumocystis carinii pneumonia

Typical Tests According to Textbook: Chest x-ray, sputum for culture, bronchoalveolar lavage.

Ira Bradley's Tests: Chest x-ray and a sputum for culture was ordered.

Kaposi's sarcoma

Typical Tests According to Textbook: Biopsy of lesions.

Ira Bradley's Tests: Nothing was ordered.

Candida (oral candidiasis)

Typical Tests According to Textbook: Scrapings of lesions for microscopic examination.

Ira Bradley's Tests: Scrapings were obtained.

Treatment (Medications)

Pneumocystis carinii pneumonia

Typical Treatment According to Textbook: Many medications listed—most common are trimethoprim and sulfamethoxazole.

Ira Bradley's Treatment: Trimethoprim and sulfamethoxazole.

Kaposi's sarcoma

Typical Treatment According to Textbook: Chemotherapy, alpha-interferon, radiation.

Ira Bradley's Treatment: Alitretinoin gel, hydroxyurea.

Candida **(oral candidiasis)**

Typical Treatment According to Textbook: Fluconazole, nystatin, clotrimazole, itroconazole, amphotericin B

Ira Bradley's Treatment: Fluconazole

4. Ira Bradley was diagnosed with HIV infection 11 years ago and began having significant problems with opportunistic infections over the last year. He seems to fit the "typical patient" picture fairly closely.

5. The documentation reflects a progressive change from disorientation and dehydration to a state of greater orientation and improved hydration.

6. Ira Bradley has an ongoing fever. Also, his respiratory rate has continually been slightly elevated.

7. Ira Bradley's pain has not changed much—it has been between 3 and 4, located in the head and chest; described as intermittent and achy.

8.

Lab Test	Result	What Does It Reflect?
Sodium	152 (high)	Hypernatremia consistent with dehydration.
Potassium	5.7 (high)	Hyperkalemia—probably resulting from diarrhea and dehydration.
Chloride	100	Normal range.
CO_2	26	Normal range.
BUN	30 (high)	Indicates dehydration.
Creatinine	1.1	Normal range—indicates adequate kidney function.
Albumin	2.1 (low)	Indicates malnutrition syndrome.
Hemoglobin	10.2 (low)	Indicative of anemia—this is common with HIV patients. Contributes to fatigue and healing.
Hematocrit	30.6 (low)	Indicative of anemia—this is common with HIV patients. Contributes to fatigue and healing.
RBCs	3.6 (low)	Indicative of anemia—this is common with HIV patients. Contribute to fatigue and healing.
Platelets	150	Normal range, but low normal.

9. D$_5$ ½ NS @ 125 cc/hour:
   Intravenous fluid
   Still replenishing fluids since patient was dehydrated when he arrived

   AZT 1 mg/kg IVPB over 1 hour q 4 hours × 24 doses:
   Antiretroviral agent—a nucleoside reverse transcriptase inhibitor (NRTI) agent; prevents viral replication of HIV
   Administered with other agents to manage HIV infection

   Trimethoprim 300 mg and sulfamethoxazole 1.5 g IVPB q 6 hours × 16 doses:
   Antibiotic
   Treatment of *Pneumocystis carinii* pneumonia

   Delavirdine myselate 400 mg PO TID:
   Antiretroviral agent—a non-nucleoside reverse transcriptase inhibitor (NNRTI)
   Used in combination with AZT to manage HIV infection

   Saquinovir 1200 mg PO TID within 2 hours of eating:
   Antiretroviral agent—a protease inhibitor (PI) agent
   Used in management of HIV infection in combination with other agents

   Fluconazole 100 mg PO AM × 14 days:
   Antifungal agent
   Used to treat candidiasis infection in mouth

   Alitretinoin gel 0.1% apply to lesions BID:
   Treatment of Kaposi's sarcoma

   Hydroxyurea:
   Antineoplastic agent
   Treatment of Kaposi's sarcoma

10. Administering antiretroviral drugs from different drug groups is an advantage because combination therapy decreases the likelihood of drug resistance.

11. There are no special precautions ordered. The nurse should follow Standard Precautions—prevention of contact with blood and body fluids. Handwashing is necessary to prevent spread of infections to all patients. The nurse should be concerned about Ira Bradley's susceptibility to infection due to immunosuppression.

12. d
13. a
14. d
15. c
16. b

Lesson 11 – HIV—Part II

1. Patient: Ira Bradley
   Room #: 309
   Age: 43
   Diagnosis: Laceration to head; AIDS; PC pneumonia; Kaposi's on leg
   Vitals: "Stable" with temp around 101 degrees
   O$_2$ Sat: 88%–89% on RA
   Pain: Not given
   Treatments: None given

Significant Assessment Findings: Awake, alert, and oriented; crackles bilaterally; difficulty swallowing from thrush with decreased PO intake; does not like wearing NC but wears when SOB; Kaposi's lesion on left thigh

IV Location/Date: Changed from L forearm to R forearm last night

Identified Patient/Family Problems: Problem with adequate intake due to difficulty swallowing. Other main problem is caregiver role strain; wife concerned about her husband.

2. Answers will vary significantly—there is not really a right or wrong answer. It may have been helpful to have an oral intake amount as well as an output amount, since the patient is not taking fluids well. It may have also been good to know about his pain status, what was given on the previous shift, and whether this helped.

3. | **Routine Medications, dose, route** | **Time Due** |
   | --- | --- |
   | AZT 1 mg/kg IVPB over 1 hour q4h × 24 doses | 0800
1200 |
   | Trimethoprim 300 mg and sulfamethoxazole 1.5 g IVPB q6h × 16 doses | 1300 |
   | Delavirdine Myselate 400 mg PO TID | 0900
1300 |
   | Saquinovir 1200 mg PO TID within 2 hours of eating | 0900
1300 |
   | Fluconazole 100 mg PO AM × 14 days | 0800 |
   | Alitretinoin gel 0.1%, apply to lesions BID | 0900 |

   No PRN medications were given.

4. Blood Pressure: 110/80
   Pulse: 84
   Respiration: 20
   Temperature: 99.8° F
   Oxygen Saturation: 92% room air
   Pain Location: Chest/throat
   Pain Characteristics: Dull achy; burning
   Level of Pain: 6

5. No

6. This is important because the saturation level is affected by the use of supplemental oxygen. The nurse should always indicate the amount of oxygen a patient is receiving when documenting oxygen saturation. If the patient is on room air, this should be indicated.

7. Pain related to inflammation of body tissue as manifested by verbalization of dull achy pain in chest and burning pain in throat and pain level of 6/10.

   Check the MAR to see what can be given and what was given last.

   Could offer either morphine or oxycodone hydrochloride as well as alternative therapies for pain management.

8. Head/Neck
   The abnormal findings are tenderness with palpation of the lymph nodes; white plaques on tongue.

   Thorax and Upper Extremities
   Crackles auscultated bilaterally; decreased expansion of chest; increased fremitus at bases.

   Abdomen and Lower Extremities
   No abnormal findings.

9. Upper extremities: IV is in the right forearm. Nurse should always include IV site assessment as part of bedside examination.

   Lower extremities: Nurse should have looked at left thigh to evaluate lesions associated with Kaposi's sarcoma.

10. a. Fluconazole

    b. This is ordered by the physician as an everyday dose. It is important that the dose is administered the same time each day, but the specific time is unimportant. If the medication was administered yesterday at 0800 and today at 0900, that is 1 hour late, but it is not considered a critical amount of time.

    c. Since it is printed on the MAR as an 0800 dose, the nurse should put a line though the 0800 and write 0900 and initial the dose.

    d. Ideally, the nurse should call pharmacy and ask them to list the medication on the MAR as an 0900 dose so that it is given at the same time as the other oral medications.

11. a. Alitretinoin Gel

    b. Ointments and gels are usually kept with other medications, although occasionally these might be kept in the patient's room at the beside or in one of the drawers of the beside table. Hospital policies vary from agency to agency; therefore do not assume this is done in all facilities.

    c. There are two likely reasons we did not see the nurse give this medication: either the patient or his wife will apply the gel or it may be applied during hygiene care.

12. Perception/Self-Concept: Feels hopeless. Focus is on sickness and dying. Not feeling ability to be independent.

    Activity: Feeling fatigued all the time. Needs to stop and rest a lot.

    Sexuality/Reproduction: Lack of sexual relations at this point; patient states no problems; wife states they are still close.

    Culture: Jewish; increased spirituality.

    Nutrition/Metabolic: Teeth OK. Patient is vegetarian. Loss of appetite; difficulty eating due to infection in mouth; has had weight loss.

    Sleep/Rest: Sleeps "all the time"; not rested at the hospital—better at home. Infections make him sleep poorly; no energy.

Role/Relationship: Close family, but illness has caused problems for the kids. Marital relationship described as close; "still love each other." Loss of friends ("seem to disappear"). Not much outside interaction since not working much.

Health Perception: Hopeless about well-being. Would like to prevent infections but does not feel he can prevent anything. Is very interested in working with an HIV coordinator to improve condition.

Elimination: BMs very unpredictable; has frequent diarrhea, especially when he has infections. Multiple UTIs.

Cognitive/Perceptual: Tired—hard to focus on conversation.

Coping/Stress: Family problems; feeling overwhelmed trying to stick together. Patient indicates he is dying—mostly just tired.

Values/Beliefs: Used to be spiritual and meditate; now he just wants to sleep. Values a good day when he can get out of bed. Not very religious. Living a little longer is important to him.

13. Ira Bradley and his family are experiencing social stigma problems at this point. Family stress and social isolation, dependency, loss of control, and economic pressures are also evident. Diarrhea is an ongoing problem. Fatigue is described as a common symptom in the textbook. Ira Bradley is experiencing fatigue as well.

14. Listed below are some acceptable answers, but these are not the only correct answers—several others are possible. What is most important is to recognize that there are many problems and to identify data to support the problems.

Nursing Diagnoses

Altered health maintenance
Ineffective management of therapeutic regime (family)
Risk for infection
Fluid volume deficit
Altered nutrition: less than body requirements
Altered oral mucous membrane
Impaired skin integrity
Impaired swallowing
Diarrhea
Activity intolerance
Fatigue
Impaired gas exchange
Sleep pattern disturbance
Chronic pain
Hopelessness
Risk for death anxiety
Risk for caregiver role strain
Altered family processes
Social isolation
Altered sexuality patterns
Ineffective individual coping
Risk for spiritual distress

Collaborative Problems

PC: Cryptococcal meningitis
PC: Cytomegaloviris
PC: Mycobacterium avium complex
PC: Wasting syndrome
PC: AIDS dementia complex

15. Answers will vary depending on the problems chosen.

Lesson 12 – Cancer

1. Initiation: The first stage of cancer—it is an irreversible alteration in cell's genetic structure.

   Promotion: Proliferation of the altered cell.

   Progression: Increased growth rate of a group of cells becomes a tumor; progression stage is characterized by increased growth rate of the tumor.

2. TAAs appear on the cell surface of malignant cells; lymphocytes continually check cell surface antigens and detect and destroy cells with TAAs.

3. Cytotoxic T cells: These play a role in resisting growth; kill tumor cells and indirectly help to stimulate T cells, natural killer cells, and B lymphocytes.

   Natural killer cells (NK): These cells directly lyse tumor cells spontaneously without prior sensitization.

   Macrophages: These play a big role, including phagocytosis of cancer cells and release of biologic response modifiers such as colony-stimulating factors, tumor necrosis factor, interleukin-1, and α-interferon.

   B-lymphocytes: These produce specific antibodies that bind to tumor cells and kill cells by complement fixation and lysis.

4. This is a malignant neoplasm that may appear as lesions on the skin or the GI tract or in a lymphoadenopathic form. In HIV, lesions may be few or multiple, and they may occur on the skin, mucous membranes, lymph nodes, and viscera.

5. Ira Bradley has immunosuppression secondary to HIV infection. He has Kaposi's sarcoma of the skin.

6. Notes from Admissions Profile: Only information found in Admissions Profile is that Kaposi's sarcoma is one of many admitting diagnoses.

7. Notes from Physical & History Section:
   Very little is noted in the Physical & History or the physicians' orders concerning the Kaposi's sarcoma.
   Emergency Department Report indicates presence of Kaposi's sarcoma on left thigh.
   Physical & History indicates Kaposi's sarcoma on left thigh.
   No indication of current or recent treatment.

8. **Orders for Ira Bradley**
   Physicians' orders: mention of Alitretinoin gel 0.1%—apply directly to lesions (following instruction sheet) BID.
   Hydroxyurea 1500 mg PO QD

   Treatment According to Textbook
   Treatment with cancer chemotherapy, alpha interferon, or radiation.

9. Palliation

10.

Nursing Diagnosis	Applicable As Is?	Suggested Modification
Altered oral mucous membrane related to chemotherapy or radiation	No	Change "related to chemotherapy or radiation" to "related to opportunistic infection."
Fatigue related to effects of cancer	Yes	None
Ineffective individual coping related to depression secondary to diagnosis and treatment	Yes	None
Body-image disturbance related to hair loss, disfiguring surgery, and weight loss	No	Data does not support this diagnosis.
Altered family processes related to cancer diagnosis of family member	No	Change "related to cancer diagnosis" to "related to AIDS diagnosis."

Lesson 13 – Fluid and Electrolyte Imbalance—Part I: Preclinical Preparation

1. **Emergency Department Report**
   Has had very little to eat or drink
   Disorientation
   Significantly underweight
   Dry mucosa
   Skin tenting
   Probable candidiasis infection of the oropharynx
   Respiratory rate 23/minute

   Physical & History
   Respiratory rate 23/min
   Temp 100.2° F
   Frequent bouts of diarrhea
   History of poor appetite
   Difficulty swallowing—painful
   Entered hospital in dehydrated state
   Plaques evident on oral mucous membrane, gums, and tongue

2. Candidiasis infection of the mouth led to decreased food/fluid intake because of the pain with swallowing. He also has pneumonia and a fever. A rapid respiratory rate and a fever increase insensible loss.

3. Subjective Data: Statements made by patient suggesting confusion
   Objective Data: Oral mucosa dry, numerous white plaques

4. Na^+: Elevated
   K^+: Normal to elevated
   Cl^-:　　Normal to elevated
   BUN: Elevated
   Creatinine: Normal (assuming normal renal function)
   Albumin: Elevated
   Hgb: Normal
   Hct: Elevated

5. IV D_5 0.45 NS @ 125 cc/hour
   Intake and output

6.

Lab	Value	L, H, N	Meaning
Na^+	152	H	Hypernatremia is associated with dehydration.
K^+	5.7	H	Hyperkalemia can occur with dehydration. Levels may also be elevated with severe infection.
Cl^-	100	N	
CO_2	26	N	
BUN	30	H	Can indicate renal function and hydration status. If elevated with normal creatinine, it is most likely attributed to dehydration. If elevated in conjunction with creatinine, it most likely points to renal problems.
Creatinine	1.1	N	Normal renal function. Validates BUN as hydration marker.
Albumin	2.1	L	Albumin levels tend to increase in presence of dehydration. However, this patient has had poor nutritional status for quite some time, so the low level can best be explained by the nutritional deficit.
Hgb	10.2	L	He is anemic, probably from nutritional deficiencies.
Hct	30.6	L	Dehydration can cause elevated levels. However, he is anemic, probably from nutritional deficiency and chronic condition.
Urine Specific Gravity	1.040	N	One would expect this level to be elevated with dehydration (above 1.030).

7.

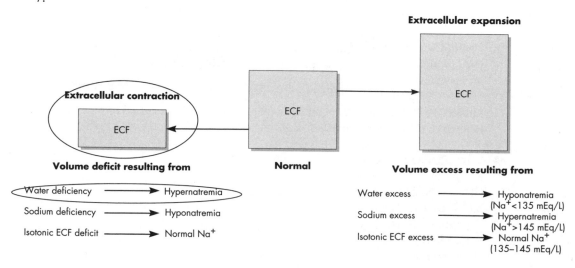

8.

Extracellular Fluid

Na$^+$ level 152

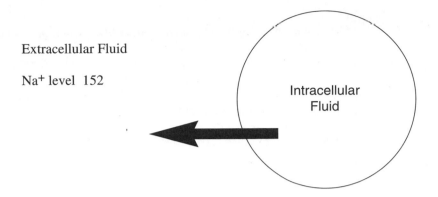

9. Treatment of underlying cause and fluid replacement.

10. **Route of fluid replacement**
Textbook: Give orally or IV
Ira Bradley's Orders: Has order for IV fluid and oral fluid

Type of IV fluid
Textbook: Dextrose solutions or hypotonic saline solution initially
Ira Bradley's Orders: D$_5$ 0.45 NaCl solution—dextrose with hypotonic saline

11. We would not expect intake to be close to output. Since Ira Bradley has cellular fluid deficits, fluids administered most likely will be absorbed, so you should not expect much urinary output.

12.

	Sunday **Admission to 2400**	**Sunday 2400 to** **Monday 0800**	**Monday** **0800 to 1600**	**Totals**
Intake Totals	500	1400	1540	3440
Output Totals	300	900	1350	2550

13. The output totals are expected when you consider the history and lab values. The intake is expected given an IV at 125 cc/hour. The output is low for a well-hydrated person, but not for someone who is recovering from dehydration. You could expect outputs to be low because he should be retaining fluid for cellular hydration and because he continues to have a fever and increased respiratory rate, thus an increased insensible loss.

14. Very little has been documented that reflects the hydration status of Ira Bradley. Only two things can be found: (1) documentation that he does not have edema and (2) documentation regarding his skin, indicating the skin is hot and dry on Sunday through Monday morning, after which it is documented as "within normal limits." This documentation is limited— other things such as skin turgor and mucous membranes should have been included.

15. **Physicians' Notes:**
Monday: Patient started on fluid repletion.
Tuesday: Stable and improving; BUN 24; creatinine 1.0; urine specific gravity 1.018.
    Dehydration is decreasing in response to fluids.

Physicians' Orders
Monday: Orders on Monday reflect continuing to monitor fluid and electrolyte status with the Chem 7 and UA order.
Tuesday: Orders do not reflect fluid and electrolyte status.

Nurses' Notes

Monday: Objective data documentation states oral mucosa is pink and dry; analysis and assessment states dehydration and that patient is now oriented to person and place.

Tuesday: Objective data documentation states he is now oriented × 3 and "rehydrating as indicated by physical assessment and lab results." IV patent: analysis and assessment state that he is "rehydrating slowly." This documentation does not seem to be consistent with the lab results or the data documented.

Lesson 14 – Fluid and Electrolyte Imbalance—Part II

1. Minimal data discussed regarding fluid/electrolyte status. Indication that IV was changed because of painful IV site. Indication of output from last shift (1450 cc), but no indication of intake. Did indicate that he is having hard time with oral fluid intake.

2. D_5 0.45 NaCl @ 125 cc/hour

3. D_5 is an isotonic fluid; 0.45 NaCl is a hypotonic saline fluid. This fluid has a hydrating effect on the body because the dextrose is metabolized, leaving free water for cellular hydration.

4. 42 gtts/minute

5. 1200 hours

6.

Assessment findings related to fluid/electrolyte status	**How do findings relate to fluid/electrolyte assessment?**
Mental status—although not formally documented, one could tell he was awake and alert, behavior appropriate.	Change in mental status is one common sign of fluid and electrolyte imbalance.
JVD was checked—was found to be not distended.	This indicates he does not have vascular fluid overload.
Oral cavity was checked. The mucous membranes were pink with presence of white plaque. Although not documented, the mucous membranes were moist.	Plaque in mouth suggests ongoing problem with infection—suggests oral intake may still be low. Moist mucous membranes indicate improved hydration status.
Grips were checked—found to be equal and weak. Also, foot strength was checked.	Muscle weakness is a common finding associated with fluid and electrolyte imbalance.
Auscultated heart—documentation of normal S_1 and S_2 without a split.	Cardiac conduction is affected by electrolyte levels, particularly potassium.
Palpated for edema—no edema found.	Edema is an indication of extracellular fluid volume excess.
Auscultated bowel sounds—documentation of normoactive bowel sounds.	Electrolyte imbalances can cause hyperactive or hypoactive sounds. Also, paralytic ileus may be related to electrolyte levels.

7. Skin turgor; IV site assessment.

8. Fluid volume deficit related to decreased fluid intake as manifested by dry mucous membranes, dry skin, decreased urine output.

9. a. Ask Ira Bradley about fluid preferences.
   Offer cool, as opposed to hot, fluids.
   Offer small-volume, frequent fluids.
   Set a goal with patient to drink a certain amount of fluid every 30 minutes.

   b. These all contribute to increased insensible loss. It is important not only to provide fluids but also to minimize insensible losses for this patient.

   c. Monitoring I&O and labs (specifically Na^+, K^+, specific gravity). Physical findings include improvement in mental status, weight gain, condition of skin and mucous membranes, and perhaps normalization of vital signs.

10.

Day	Data	Source
Tuesday	• Tolerating liquids with no nausea or vomiting.	Physicians' notes
	• Decrease IV fluid rate to 75 cc/hour.	Physicians' orders
	• Tolerating regular diet; shows improvement in appetite.	Nurses' notes
Wednesday	• Tolerating liquids and solid foods—repeat labs for tomorrow morning.	Physicians' notes
	• Order for a UA and Chem 7.	Physicians' orders
	• Indication of increased oral intake.	Nurses' notes
Thursday	• Scheduled for discharge tomorrow; thrush resolving; eating and drinking with no nausea or vomiting. Labs given.	Physicians' notes
	• DC IV.	Physicians' orders
	• Morning discharge.	Nurses' notes

11.

Test	Sunday	Tuesday	Thursday
Na^+	152	148	142
K^+	5.7	5.2	4.8
Cl^-	100	100	100
CO_2	26	26	26
BUN	30	24	18.1
Creatinine	1.1	1.0	1.0
Urine specific gravity	1.040	1.025	1.018

Explanation for changes: Sodium and potassium levels, as well as urine specific gravity, decrease in response to the IV fluids for rehydration. The BUN is initially high, probably in response to dehydration—this level also decreases with hydration.

12.

	Intake Totals	Output Totals
Sunday	500	200
Monday	4440	2150
Tuesday	5800	5360
Wednesday	4740	4500
Thursday	3530	2700

Explanation: During the first 24 to 48 hours of admission, it would appear that Ira Bradley is retaining fluids because his output is so much less than his input. However, the output is reduced because he is rehydrating—fluid is shifting back into the cells.

13. Sara Terney: Indicates the need to explore ongoing treatment of oral candidiasis.

Ray Burns: Refers to the problems associated with oral candidiasis and adverse effects on Ira Bradley. Specifically, he addresses the need for adequate hydration and the potential need for rehydration on a regular basis (because of fever and dehydration).

Bridget Natalicio: Nothing mentioned.

14. Family needs to understand how fluid loss occurs quickly and to be aware of things they can do at home to prevent dehydration. Comfort measures for the mouth will go a long way. Recording amount of fluid intake during the day may also maintain an awareness before dehydration occurs.

Lesson 15 – Perioperative Care

1. 1530 hours

2. 1615 hours

3. Elective

4. a. Health care provider must adequately disclose the diagnosis or condition.
   Patient must be able to have sufficient comprehension of the information.
   Patient must give consent voluntarily.

   b. It is documented that David Ruskin was oriented only to person—he was not oriented to time, place, or the situation. In this case, he was not legally cognitively oriented to understand the surgical consent form.

5. None of these fears were documented in the Emergency Department Report. Often, especially when the procedure is urgent in nature, issues that are not life-threatening are not well explored or documented.

6. The most important thing to note is that there is really no documented preop assessment in David Ruskin's chart. The Physical & History documented in the chart was done after the surgery. A preoperative assessment should always be done before all surgeries, even emergency surgery. With emergency surgery, this assessment will typically be brief compared with a more thorough assessment for planned surgery.

7. David Ruskin and his wife should have been told a little bit about the surgical procedure, the expected length of surgery, and perhaps most important, what to expect after surgery, such as mobility and pain issues. Although David Ruskin was initially disoriented when he arrived in the ER, his Glasgow Coma Scale was at 15 shortly before surgery, so he and his wife could have benefited from teaching.

8. Benzodiazepines and barbiturates: Sedative and amnesic properties

   Anticholinergics: Reduce secretions

   Narcotics: Decrease intraoperative anesthetic requirement and analgesia

   Antiemetics: Decrease nausea and vomiting

   Antibiotics: Prophylactic treatment of infection

   Low dose heparin: Decrease incidence of deep vein thrombosis

9. David Ruskin received narcotics and antibiotics before surgery.

10. 1640 hours

11. Anesthesia at 1700; incision at 1710.

12. Open reduction, internal fixation

13. Insertion of rod into the humerus; fixation of two posterior shaft segments with screws.

14. 1850

15. Respiratory and circulatory adequacy; assessment of the surgical site; pain.

16. Airway obstruction after anesthesia is most often caused by blockage from the patient's tongue. Hypoxemia is most often caused by atelectasis.

17. Patient awake
    Vital signs stable
    No excess bleeding or drainage
    Oxygen saturation >90%
    Report to receiving floor given

18. Table 15-1   Nursing Assessment and Care of Patient on Admission to Clinical Unit

---

✓ • Record time of patient's return to unit
✓ • Take baseline vital signs
      Assess airway and breath sounds
✓ • Assess neurologic status, including level of consciousness and movement of extremities
✓ • Assess wound, dressing, drainage tubes
      Note type and amount of drainage
      Connect tubing to gravity or suction drainage
  • Assess color and appearance of skin
  • Assess urinary status
      Note time of voiding
      Note presence of catheter and total output
      Check for bladder distention or urge to void
      Note catheter patency

- Assess pain and discomfort
    - Note last dose and type of pain control
    - Note current pain intensity
✓ - Position for airway maintenance, comfort, safety (bed in low position, side rails up)
- Check IV infusion
    - Note type of solution
    - Note amount of fluid remaining
    - Note flow rate
    - Check integrity of insertion site and size of catheter
- Attach call light within reach and reorient patient to use of call light
- Ensure that emesis basin and tissues are available
- Determine emotional condition and support
    - Check for presence of family member or significant other
✓ - Check and carry out postoperative orders

19. Pain
    Risk for infection
    Anxiety
    Risk for constipation
    PC: Thromboembolism
    PC: Hemorrhage
    PC: Urinary retention

20. This list will probably vary considerably from student to student, but it should include post-op complications with neurovascular compromise and safety (given the fact that he has a CHI).

Lesson 16 – Pneumonia—Part I: Preclinical Preparation

1. Respiratory distress, fever, R/O Hantavirus versus pneumonia.

2. Symptoms include fatigue, SOB, malaise, feels hot × 2 days. Increased cough, sick to her stomach and decreased appetite for 3–4 days.

3. MI 5 years ago
   Congestive heart failure
   Angina
   COPD—chronic bronchitis
   Hypertension

4. A virus that is capable of causing hemorrhagic fever or pneumonia leading to massive pulmonary edema and respiratory failure. Transmission to humans is believed to be from close contact with the droppings of infected rodents.

5. Sally Begay reported cleaning out a barn 1 week ago—states she saw mouse droppings in the barn. She also reportedly did not wear a mask when cleaning the barn.

6. Community-acquired pneumonia

7. Congestion: Organisms cause fluid shift into the alveoli. Organisms multiply in the serous fluid and the infection spreads. Bacteria damages the host by overwhelming growth to point of interfering with lung function.

   Red hepatization: Massive dilation of the capillaries—alveoli are filled with organisms, neutrophils, RBCs, and fibrin. Lung appears red and granular.

Gray hepatization: Blood flow decreases—leukocytes and fibrin consolidate in the affected part of the lung.

Resolution: Resolution and healing occur—exudate becomes lysed and is processed by macrophages. Normal lung tissue is restored and gas-exchange ability returns to normal.

8.

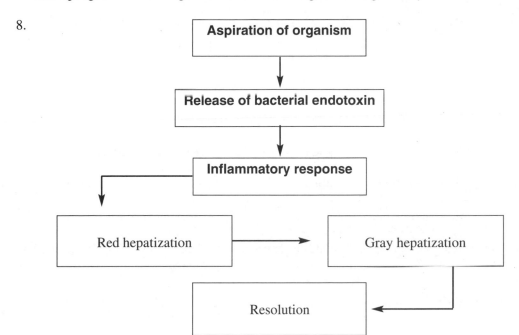

9. The correct answer is choice e (COPD—chronic bronchitis).

10. X History and physical examination   X ABG

    X Chest x-ray   X CBC

    X Gram's stain of sputum   X Blood cultures

    X Sputum culture

11. Alveolar infiltrate in the right middle and lower lung. The other findings are consistent with chronic bronchitis.

12.

Test	Normal Value	Sally Begay's results
Hgb	12–16 g/dl	13.3
Hct	38%–47%	40.1
WBC	4.0–11.0	32.9
RBC	4.0–5.0	4.32
Platelets	150–400	166

13.

Test	Normal Value	Sally Begay's results
pH	7.35–7.45	7.37
$PaCO_2$	35–45	43
PaO_2	75–100	87
HCO_3	20–30	23

14. The CBC tells us that Sally Begay has a severe bacterial infection—we know this because of the elevated WBC. The ABG tells us that even though she is experiencing shortness of breath, Sally Begay has adequate oxygen exchange.

15.

Medication	Type/Classification	Role in Treatment of Pneumonia
Erythromycin	Antibiotic	Treatment of her infection
Ceftizoxime	Antibiotic	Treatment of her infection
Acetaminophen	Analgesia/antipyretic	Treatment of fever associated with pneumonia
Albuterol	Bronchodilator	Will help dilate the airway; will enhance air movement and elimination of secretions

16. EES is for treatment of upper and lower respiratory infections; bacteriostatic action with spectrum against many gram-positive cocci and bacilli, as well as gram-negative pathogens.

Ceftizoxime is a third-generation cephalosporin that has bactericidal action; useful for treatment of respiratory tract infection.

It is not uncommon for two antibiotics to be ordered for severe infections so that they exert the same therapeutic effect, but go about it in different ways.

17. 0900   Hydroclorothiazide 25 mg PO
            Potassium chloride 10 mEq PO q am
            Digoxin 0.125 mg PO

    1200   Albuterol IPPB (given by RT)

    1400   Ceftizoxime 1 gram IVBP

18. Erythromycin was originally ordered to be given 500 mg IVPB q 6 hours. A new order was to discontinue the IV dose and start oral dose on a BID basis. Since the 0600 dose was given IV, the next dose of EES is not due until 1800. When in doubt, go back to the physicians' orders and read the orders there.

19. Yes, this is compatible. Most nursing drug references will include fluid compatibility for IV medications.

20. Sally Begay has been nauseated, with a loss of appetite. She also has had a fever and increased respiratory rate, thus increasing her insensible losses. She probably needs the IV fluid to keep her well hydrated while she has this infection.

Lesson 17 – Pneumonia—Part II

1. Patient: Sally Begay
   Room: 304
   Age: 68
   Diagnosis: Viral pneumonia
   Vitals: Ran temp last evening (100.4° F); afebrile on night shift; HR 87–90; RR 20–24
   O_2 Sat: 88%–89% RA
   Pain: No chest pain
   Treatments: None given
   Significant Assessment Findings: Crackles in right middle and lower lungs—otherwise clear. Productive cough, swallows sputum. Had oxygen 2 L NC on all night.
   WBC decreasing; platelets are stable.
   IV location/date: Not given
   Identified Patient/Family Problems: No problems identified.

2. Age is stated in report as 68; Sally Begay is 58. The nurse indicated that Sally Begay has viral pneumonia; however, the chart indicates she has bacterial pneumonia.

3. These are not significant errors because they do not change your nursing care. However it is important to check the records to see whether there has been inconsistent documentation in her record or on the Kardex. If inconsistencies exist, the data should be clarified.

4. Heart rate: 96

   Blood pressure: (150/98)

   Temperature: (99.9)

   Respiratory rate: 20

   Oxygen saturation: 93%

   Pain: (5 to 6/10) Pain is achy—located in chest.

5. Sally Begay is wearing nail polish. This potentially can cause inaccurate measurement of the oxygen saturation. Ideally, the nail polish should be removed on the finger used to place the probe.

6. The temperature indicates low-grade fever; probably not a concern requiring action. The blood pressure is high; since she has hypertension, it would be important to see what her blood pressure has been running while in the hospital. If it is a significant change or deviation, the physician should be notified. The pain is 5 to 6/10; this warrants intervention. Pain relief strategies should be explored.

7. Head and Neck: PERRLA, 3-mm pupils; oculomotor function +; facial symmetry; oral mucosa dry; full ROM to neck; no pain; no lymphadenopathy; no JVD; carotid pulse +3.

   Chest/Upper Extremities: Lungs have crackles in right lower lobes; excursion normal. S_1 and S_2; no splitting of S_2; radial pulse = +3; cap refill <3 sec; grips = strong.

   Abdomen and Lower Extremities: +BS; soft, nontender; post tib pulse +3; dorsalis pedis +2 and +3; cap refill <3 sec; no edema.

8. The most important data is the evaluation of the respiratory status—specifically lung sounds. It would have been beneficial to include respiratory effort and overall skin color as indicators of her respiratory status.

9. Perceptual/Self-Concept: Worries about things at home because husband cannot do all the work himself. Verbalizes ability to care for herself—just feels tired.

Activity: Normally works with animals at home and gets a lot of exercise. Right now, she has limitations because it is "hard to catch breath."

Sexuality/Reproduction: Menopausal; has son and two daughters. "Old now" but still close to husband.

Culture: Traditional Navajo.

Nutrition-Metabolic: No issues or significant data.

Sleep-Rest: Sleeping is "difficult"; usually feels rested after sleeping; limited energy this past week. Has been resting a lot at home.

Role/Relationship: Everyone helps each other out; many family members and friends.

Health Perception: Usually is healthy, except for the past week.

Elimination: Usually has BM daily; no BM × 2 days.

Cognitive/Perceptual: No problems; memory intact.

Coping/Stress: Family works problems out. Good support systems, but is worried about not being able to keep up at home.

Value/Belief: Sees medicine man. Family, animals, and friends are most important to her.

10. Nursing Assessment: Table 17-1   Pneumonia

Subjective Data
Important Health Information
Past health history: Lung cancer, COPD, diabetes, chronic debilitating disease, malnutrition, altered consciousness, AIDS, exposure to chemical toxins, dust, or allergens
Medications: Use of antibiotics; corticosteroids, chemotherapy, or any other immunosuppressants
Surgeries or other treatment: Recent abdominal or thoracic surgery, splenectomy, endotracheal intubation, or any surgery with general anesthesia

Functional Health Patterns
Health perception-health management: Cigarette smoking, alcoholism; recent upper respiratory tract infection, malaise
Nutritional-metabolic: Anorexia, nausea, vomiting; chills
Activity-exercise: Prolonged bed rest or immobility; fatigue, weakness, dyspnea, cough (productive or nonproductive); nasal congestion
Cognitive-perceptual: Pain with breathing, chest pain, sore throat, headache, abdominal pain, muscle aches

Objective Data
General
Fever, restlessness or lethargy; splinting of affected area

Respiratory
Tachypnea, pharyngitis; asymmetric chest movements or retraction; decreased excursion; nasal flaring; use of accessory muscles (neck, abdomen); grunting; crackles, friction rub on auscultation; dullness on percussion over consolidated areas, increased tactile fremitus on palpation; pink, rusty, purulent, green, yellow, or white sputum (amount may be scant to copious)

Cardiovascular
Tachycardia

Neurologic
Changes in mental status, ranging from confusion to delirium

Possible Findings
Leukocytosis, abnormal ABGs with decreased or normal PaO_2, decreased $PaCO_2$, and increased pH initially, and later decreased PaO_2, increased $PaCO_2$, and decreased pH; positive sputum Gram's stain and culture; patchy or diffuse infiltrates, abscesses, pleural effusion, or pneumothorax on chest x-ray

---

11. Listed below are several possible answers, but these are not the only correct answers—
    many others are possible.

Nursing Diagnoses	Collaborative Problems
Ineffective breathing pattern	PC: Hypoxemia
Impaired gas exchange	
Activity intolerance	
Hyperthermia	
Risk for altered nutrition: less than body requirements	
Fluid volume deficit	
Pain	
Fatigue	
Sleep pattern disturbance	
Constipation	
Home maintenance management impaired	

12. Answers will vary depending on which diagnoses or problems each student chooses.

13. Documentation of gradual improvement in respiratory status with notation of decreased
    need for oxygen, stabilization of oxygen saturation, vital signs, and improvement of
    appetite.

14. Nurses' notes paint a picture of gradual increase in appetite, gradual increase in activity,
    gradual improvement of oxygen exchange. Vital signs are consistent with normalization of
    vitals.

15. 4.5 days

16. 7 days

17. Probably as early as day 2; she had significant fatigue and dyspnea for several days. She
    was slow to recover even after antibiotics were started.

18. Her history of chronic bronchitis most likely caused this.

Lesson 18 – COPD

1. 10 years

2. Hypertension
   Coronary artery disease
   Myocardial infarction 5 years ago

3.
Medication	Dose	Classification of Medication and Reason Taken
Hydrochlorothiazide	25 mg qd	Diuretic—treatment of hypertension
Digoxin	0.125 mg qd	Inotropic agent
Nitroglycerin	No dose given	Vasodilator—treatment of intermittent angina pain

4. Risk for CVA—due to her ongoing history of HTN and CAD.

   Risk for DM—both parents had DM; she is Native American. Both of these increase her
   risk.

5. Chronic obstructive pulmonary disease: Disease state characterized by the presence of air-flow obstruction caused by emphysema or bronchitis—but not asthma.

   Emphysema: Enlargement of airspaces distal to the terminal bronchioles, accompanied by destruction of their walls.

   Chronic bronchitis: Presence of chronic cough for 3 months in each of 2 successive years in a patient in whom other causes of chronic cough have been excluded.

6. Cigarette smoking: This is the major risk factor; 80%–90% of COPD deaths are related to tobacco use. Cigarette smoke causes hyperplasia of cells, resulting in increased production of mucus and decreased diameter of the airway. Also reduces ciliary activity.

   Infection: Recurring respiratory tract infections contribute to aggravation and progression of COPD. These infections impair normal defense mechanisms; the multiple infections cause pathologic destruction of the lung tissue.

   Ambient air pollution: High level of air pollution is thought to cause chronic irritation to the lungs, but this is not clear.

   Heredity: A very small number of individuals have AAT genetic abnormality leading to COPD (less than 1% of all causes of COPD). Most cases are those of Northern European origin.

   Aging: Advanced age will contribute to COPD, but this alone does not typically cause COPD.

7. Chronic respiratory infection is a high probability. We know Sally Begay is currently not a smoker, but the chart is not clear about the possibility of past smoking. This is something that could easily be clarified. Although she lives in a rural area, it is possible that frequent inhalation of dust from her farm may also be a contributing factor. Additionally, many people depend on wood-burning stoves for heat and cooking on the Navajo Reservation, consequently increasing air pollution. Sally Begay is only 58 years old, so this is not the primary cause. However, at this point, her age may begin to become a factor.

8. Chronic inflammation of the lung tissue causes changes characteristic of chronic bronchitis. Inflammatory response causes vasodilation, congestion and mucosal edema. This leads to swelling and excess thick mucus, which causes narrowing of the airway lumen, resulting in diminished airflow. This increases the effort of breathing; hypoxemia and hypercapnia may develop. The mucus literally causes a physical barrier to ventilation, which interferes with oxygen diffusion. Retained mucus stimulates coughing; however the mucus cannot adequately be removed because decreased airflow into the lungs reduces the cough effort.

9. Diagrams will vary; here is one acceptable example.

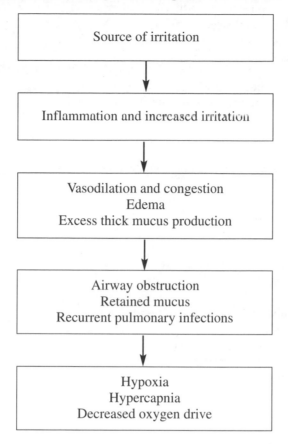

```
┌─────────────────────────────────────────┐
│          Source of irritation           │
└─────────────────────────────────────────┘
                    │
                    ▼
┌─────────────────────────────────────────┐
│     Inflammation and increased irritation │
└─────────────────────────────────────────┘
                    │
                    ▼
┌─────────────────────────────────────────┐
│        Vasodilation and congestion        │
│                  Edema                    │
│         Excess thick mucus production     │
└─────────────────────────────────────────┘
                    │
                    ▼
┌─────────────────────────────────────────┐
│            Airway obstruction             │
│              Retained mucus               │
│        Recurrent pulmonary infections     │
└─────────────────────────────────────────┘
                    │
                    ▼
┌─────────────────────────────────────────┐
│                 Hypoxia                   │
│               Hypercapnia                 │
│          Decreased oxygen drive           │
└─────────────────────────────────────────┘
```

10. Patients with chronic bronchitis are at risk for multiple pulmonary infections because of chronic inflammation and retained mucus.

11. Pleural thickening bilaterally; blunting of costophrenic angles. Increased anterior-posterior diameter of the thoracic cage.

12. Sally Begay's O_2 Sat: 87%

    Normal Range O_2 Sat: >95%

13. Oxygen saturation measurement is an indirect measurement of the percentage of well-oxygenated blood circulating, thus an indirect assessment of the oxygenation status of the patient. Her oxygen saturation is low, probably because mucus is interfering with the diffusion of oxygen in the lungs.

14. The order was for 2 liters nasal cannula. This provides oxygen concentration of about 28%.

15. Patients with chronic bronchitis or emphysema develop chronic hypercapnia. This changes the stimulus to breathe from elevated CO2 levels to low oxygen levels. Aggressive oxygen administration in these patients can result in a loss of the breathing drive.

16. The only medication ordered that specifically addresses the COPD is albuterol. Albuterol is a bronchodilator—it is helpful because it dilates the distal airways, allowing a greater diffusion of oxygen in the alveoli. It is administered via nebulizer; the advantage to administering this medication via this route is that there are few systemic effects.

17. **Identified Problems:**
Altered respiratory pattern
Altered gas exchange
Nutrition < current needs
Fatigue

Planned Interventions:
Oxygen (keep O_2 sat above 90%)
Pulmonary toilet q 2 hours
IPPB treatment
Pain medications
Activity—up in chair and ambulate TID
Rest
Oral hygiene
Monitor I&O
Monitor food intake—offer snacks

How will these be evaluated?
O_2 saturation
Lung sounds
Respiratory effort—report of less fatigue
Length of activity; distance ambulating
Condition of mucus membranes
I&O q shift/food intake
Ask about level of fatigue

18. Self-care deficit
Sleep pattern deficits

19.

Assessment Area	Saturday 1600	Tuesday 0400
Temperature	99.4° F	99.4° F
Heart rate	104	96
Respiration	24	20
Oxygen saturation	93%	93%
Use of oxygen	NC 2 L	NC 2 L
Respiratory pattern	Tachypneic	Within defined limits
Lung fields	Crackles right lower and middle lobes	Crackles right lower and middle lobes
Cough	Productive	Productive
Sputum	Unable to assess	Unable to assess

20. Not much has changed based on physical examination findings. You would want to know what the activity level has been, how much she has eaten, and what her level of fatigue is. You would also want to know how much fluid intake she has had.

21. Chest physiotherapy; push fluids to help liquefy secretions; teach effective cough techniques. Teaching pursed-lip breathing may be helpful;

22. Rose Simpson, RN
    Nurse Case Manager

    Needs patient education. Concerned about health care needs in rural area. Has limited access to regular health care.

    Concerned about lack of culturally sensitive interventions.

    Need for educational outreach and attempts to find access to health care and community nursing.

    Louise Johnson, RN
    Clinical Nurse Specialist

    Concerned about multiple conditions (MI, HTN, and COPD) and her risk for continued respiratory infections.

    Need for educational outreach with specific focus on how to prevent respiratory infections.

    Possibly recommend pneumonia and flu vaccines.

    Kris Holmes, MSW
    Social Worker

    Concerned about multiple chronic problems and adequate health care access. Need for strong educational outreach program.

    Another issue is social support; involvement of others who help the family.

    Cultural issues need to be addressed; need to develop culturally sensitive health care.

23. What is very consistent is the concern all three had for education. The textbook clearly indicates that the most important aspect in long-term care of patients with COPD is education. This is very consistent and an obvious priority.

    The biggest physical concern probably is her respiratory infection.

    The biggest challenge is the cultural diversity issue.

Lesson 19 – Hypertension

1. The force of blood exerted against the walls of the blood vessel.

2. Arterial blood pressure = cardiac output × systemic vascular resistance

    Interpretation: Mechanisms that regulate BP can affect either CO or SVR or both. Regulation is complex, involving nervous, cardiovascular, renal, and endocrine function. SVR is the resistance in blood flow—usually exerted by the diameter of the blood vessels. The greater the resistance, the greater the BP.

3.

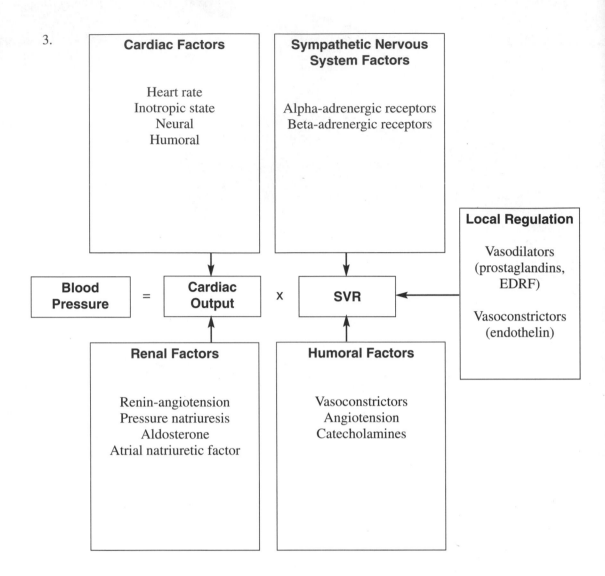

4. Baroreceptors are located in the carotid artery and arch of the aorta. They are specialized nerve cells that are sensitive to stretch; with increased BP there is increased stretch. When these are stretched, they send a signal to the brainstem, which then causes an inhibition of sympathetic activity. This reduced SNS activity decreases heart rate, decreases force of contraction, and causes vasodilation in the peripheral blood vessels. All of these result in a drop in BP. When there is a loss of stretch (associated with hypotension), the baroreceptors send a signal to the brainstem, which then causes a stimulation of sympathetic activity.

5. 5 years

6. 163/92

7. Medication: Hydrochlorothiazide

   Dose: 25 mg qd

   Classification of Medication: Diuretic

8. Sustained elevation of BP—(SBP is ≥140 and DBP is ≥90) for extended periods of time. Diagnosis is made if BP is elevated on more than three occasions during several weeks.

9. Hypertension typically causes no symptoms unless the BP is very high—then the patient may complain of a headache

10. She would be experiencing stage 2 hypertension with SBP >160 and DBP >90

11. Age
    Sex
    Family history
    (We do not know enough based on data provided to comment on serum lipids, sodium intake, or the socioeconomic status. She is somewhat active on the farm tending the animals, so sedentary lifestyle probably did not contribute to this. She is 5'6" and weighs 150 pounds. Although she is overweight, she is not obese. She does not smoke or drink alcohol.)

12. Sally Begay indicates she lives a distance from town, which could interfere with her ability to follow health care advice and/or medication schedule.

    When asked about her usually blood pressure, Sally Begay indicates she is "not sure, but thinks it is OK." This statement may be an indication that she is not having her blood pressure monitored on a regular basis.

    Sally Begay indicates she has no dietary restrictions. Further clarification would be appropriate because she may have been prescribed a low-salt diet.

    Sally Begay describes self as Traditional Navajo and "likes to see the medicine man as well as the regular doctor." This information could be an important lead into her beliefs about taking medication, particularly for a disease she cannot feel. Need to consider whether past recommendations have been culturally sensitive.

13. Primary: Primary hypertension accounts for 95% of all cases. Cause is unknown but is thought to be associated with multiple factors, including SNS stimulation, obesity, lipid levels, sodium intake, etc.

    Secondary: Secondary hypertension accounts for only 5% of all cases. Causes are multiple, but cause can be specifically identified; for example, narrowing of the aorta, endocrine disorder, head injury, side effect from medications, etc.

14. Most likely, Sally Begay has primary hypertension; the secondary causes do not seem to be consistent with her history.

15. Yes. She has already had a myocardial infarction a few years ago.

16. She belongs in risk group C because she has at least one TOD and has stage 2 HTN.

17. This is a way of classifying the amount of risk individuals with HTN have for CV disease. These factors partly indicate the type of treatment that is recommended.

18-20.

Diagnostic Test	How Test Might Help Identify TOD	Results
Chest x-ray	May show evidence of an enlarged heart	Does not indicate heart is enlarged
BUN	Information about renal function	16 (normal finding)
Creatinine	Information about renal function	1 (normal finding)
EKG monitoring	Information about cardiac conduction	Normal sinus rhythm— normal finding

21. Saturday 1600: 158/90
    Saturday 2400: 156/88
    Sunday 0800: 155/86
    Sunday 1600: 152/84
    Sunday 2400: 152/81
    Monday 0800: 148/82
    Monday 1600: 147/81
    Monday 2400: 150/82
    Tuesday 0800: 152/78
    Tuesday 1600: 146/76
    Tuesday 2400: 142/78
    Wednesday 0800: 144/73
    Wednesday 1600: 146/76
    Wednesday 2400: 142/74
    Thursday 0800: 143/76
    Thursday 1600: 148/77
    Thursday 2400: 140/72

22. The SBP and the DBP both come down gradually between Monday and Thursday. There are two possible explanations, one being she gradually has less effort breathing and less fever. A second possibility is a compliance issue with the medication she is taking—Does she take it consistently at home? What are her beliefs about the medication?

23. Ideally, the goal BP will be consistently below 140/90. Although her diastolic pressure is down, the systolic is higher than target goal.

    Also, she is currently taking a diuretic, but since she has previously had an MI, she really should be on a beta-blocker and perhaps an ACE inhibitor.

24. First and foremost is the need to do a cultural assessment and to assess her level of understanding about her hypertension. Based on this information, you will have a better idea in what areas she needs teaching. Finally, assess her style of learning—How does she learn best?

25. The teaching plan will vary considerably from student to student. However, here is some information that should be included: instruction regarding the medications, her thoughts about taking the medication, and a discussion about some side effects; potential dangers of uncontrolled hypertension; the need for ongoing monitoring of BP. You should perhaps explore possibility of patient's family learning to take BP at home and keeping a record so that this can be evaluated by physician when she goes to the clinic.

Lesson 20 – Coronary Artery Disease

1. U Age   U Family history

   M Elevated serum lipids   M Smoking

   M Inactivity   M Hypertension

   M Obesity   U Race

   U Gender   M Stress/behavior patterns

2. Chest pain caused by cardiac ischemia.

3. Myocardial ischemia develops when the demand for oxygen exceeds the ability of the coronary arteries to supply it. The oxygen supply is depleted because of insufficient blood flow, a result of narrowing of the arteries.

4. Answers can be any of the following:
   Physical exertion
   Strong emotions
   Eating a large meal
   Temperature extremes
   Cigarette smoking
   Sexual activity
   Stimulants
   Circadian rhythm

5. She has not had angina in over a year.

6. Sally Begay has nitroglycerin at home. Nitroglycerin causes vasodilation of the coronary arteries, thereby increasing blood flow and oxygen to the cardiac muscle.

7. Stable angina

8. An MI is irreversible damage to myocardial cells caused by lack of oxygen. Necrosis of the tissue occurs in the area where there is a loss of oxygenated blood. Loss of blood flow is usually due to a thrombosis within one of the coronary arteries, thus blocking flow of blood. The more cardiac tissue affected, the greater the area of heart tissue that dies. One usually has a sudden onset of severe crushing-like chest pain. The pain is due to a loss of oxygenated blood flow to the cardiac tissue.

9. Uncontrolled hypertension is one of the leading causes of CAD, thus predisposing an individual to an MI. This may have been one of the major causes of Sally Begay's MI 5 years ago.

10. An MI causes permanent damage to part of the heart. If the damage is significant enough, cardiac output is affected, and often the patient is at risk for, or actually develops, CHF. It is also possible that the CHF is a consequence of uncontrolled hypertension.

11. Much information in this section is consistent with Sally Begay's history. First, her age is a factor. She manifested the disease 5 years ago, making her 53 at the time. Sally Begay has periodic symptoms of angina as well as having an MI. In postmenopausal women, hypertension is associated with a higher incidence of CAD.

12. The cardiac monitoring is simply a precaution, most likely ordered because of her past history of MI, CABG, CHF, and HTN. The monitor displays the electrical impulse of the heart. It is useful in early recognition of cardiac dysrhythmia.

13. The nurse should include the cardiac rhythm as part of the routine documentation.

14. Nurses have documented that she is in normal sinus rhythm.

15. Pain from angina is usually located in the same general area as pain from an MI; however it tends to be considered "mild to moderate" and typically lasts up to 15 minutes. Also, angina usually is relieved with rest and/or nitroglycerin. Pain from an MI is more severe in nature, has a sudden onset, lasts from a half-hour to several hours and is unrelieved by rest or nitroglycerin.

   Chest pain from pneumonia is very different from angina or MI pain. Although the pain may be located in the chest, it typically is described as dull. Patient will have a cough and fever. Pain often increases with coughing.

16. Answers will vary depending on how selective students are when recording data. The most important things to include:
    - Nutrition data (does not like sweets; prefers cheese and mutton; may have milk intolerance; eats fruit and vegetables "occasionally")
    - Cultural data (traditional Navajo)
    - Usually self sufficient, but right now is fatigued easily

17. Probably need to further explore types of foods eaten, who prepares the meals, how foods are selected, what family members are typically present at mealtime. Also, it is very important to explore her beliefs and values regarding dietary modification for control of disease.

18. Cheese and mutton are her foods of preference; both are very high in fat. Based on the interview data, it seems that Sally Begay does not eat many fruits/vegetables. The sample menus in Table 32-5 are low-fat meals, in which vegetables/fruits appear frequently.

19. Although this table is very helpful for ideas, it would be unrealistic to expect that it is culturally sensitive to a middle-age Navajo woman. It would be useful from the standpoint of getting ideas for suggesting which types of food she should try to eat and which types of foods she should try to restrict. It is vital that students understand that modifications to the sample menu would need to be made or it is unlikely it would be appealing to Sally Begay (a very "American food" diet).

Lesson 21 – Congestive Heart Failure—Part I: Tuesday

1. The correct answer is choice c.

2. The correct answer is choice b.

3. **Left-Sided Failure**

   Hypertension
   CAD
   Cardiomyopathy
   Rheumatic diseases

   Right-Sided Failure

   Left-sided failure is most common cause
   Cor pulmonale

4.

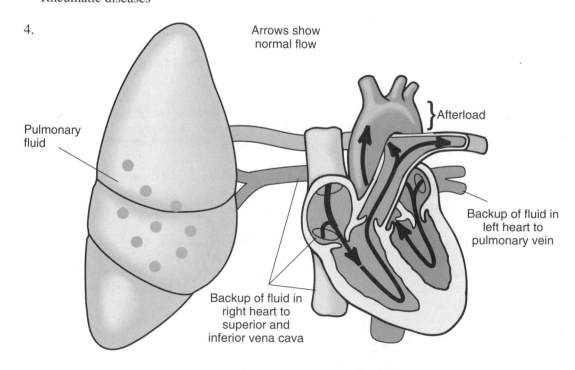

Arrows show normal flow

Afterload

Pulmonary fluid

Backup of fluid in left heart to pulmonary vein

Backup of fluid in right heart to superior and inferior vena cava

5. She does not know about medications.
   In the history, cardiopulmonary, Carmen Gonzales reports difficult breathing, fatigue, exhaustion, and increased cough, no sputum.
   In physical examination: Patient has rales in both lower lobes, poor tissue perfusion of lower extremities with cap refill >3 seconds.

6. Include indication of peripheral edema.
   She needs a current chest x-ray to determine size of heart and possibility of infiltrate because she is short of breath and tired.

7.

Risk Factors	Does Carmen Gonzales have this risk factor?	What data support your answer?
Advancing age	No	She is only 58 years old
Coronary artery disease	Yes	History
Hypertension	Yes	Vital signs: elevated BP 150/100
Diabetes	Yes	Diabetes is more likely to predispose CHF in women than in men.
Smoking	No	She is not a smoker
Obesity	Yes	She is 5'2" tall and weighs 170 pounds (BMI = 31)
Elevated cholesterol levels	No	No evidence of these lab values

8. Under Sleep and Relaxation, Carmen Gonzales reports problems sleeping, but she does not indicate exactly what this means.
   Reports difficulty breathing, fatigue,

9. There are no orders other than to monitor vitals.

10. Since congestive heart failure often manifests with respiratory symptoms, monitor oxygen saturation, breathing effort, and lung sounds. Peripheral manifestations include presence of peripheral edema and neck vein distention.

11. Temperature: 99° F   Respiration: 24

    Pulse: 88   Blood pressure: 150/100

    Pain rating: 8   Oxygen saturation: 91%

12. Blood pressure is too high.
    Respiration is too high.
    Temperature indicates a low grade fever.
    Pain level suggests inadequate pain control.

13. Analgesics should be given. Since you are a nursing student, you need to let the primary nurse know about the vitals. It would probably be a good idea for the nurse to notify the physician regarding the blood pressure and elevated RR. However, you would conduct bedside assessment first before calling!

14. Table 21-1   Congestive Heart Failure

Subjective Data

Important Health Information

* *Past health history:* CAD (including recent MI), hypertension, cardiomyopathy, valvular or congenital heart disease, diabetes mellitus, thyroid or lung disease, rapid or irregular heartbeat
* *Medications:* Use of and compliance with any cardiac medications; use of diuretics, estrogens, corticosteroids, phenylbutazone, nonsteroidal antiinflammatory drugs

Functional Health Patterns

* *Health perception-health management:* Fatigue
   Nutritional-metabolic: Usual sodium intake; nausea, vomiting, anorexia, stomach bloating; weight gain
* *Elimination:* Nocturia, decreased daytime urinary output, constipation
   Activity-exercise: Dyspnea, orthopnea, cough; palpitations; dizziness, fainting
* *Sleep-rest:* Number of pillows used for sleeping; paroxysmal nocturnal dyspnea
   Cognitive-perceptual: Chest pain or heaviness; RUQ pain, abdominal discomfort; behavioral changes

Objective Data

Integumentary

Cool, diaphoretic skin; cyanosis or pallor, peripheral edema (right-sided heart failure)

Respiratory

* Tachypnea, crackles, rhonchi, wheezes; frothy, blood-tinged sputum

Cardiovascular

Tachycardia, S_3, S_4, murmurs; pulsus alternans, PMI displaced inferiorly and posteriorly, jugular vein distention

Gastrointestinal

Abdominal distention, hepatosplenomegaly, ascites

Neurologic

Restlessness, confusion, decreased attention or memory

Possible Findings

Altered serum electrolytes (especially Na^+ and K^+), elevated BUN, creatinine, or liver function tests; chest x-ray demonstrating cardiomegaly, pulmonary congestion, and interstitial pulmonary edema; echocardiogram showing increased chamber size and decreased wall motion; atrial and ventricular enlargement on ECG; ↑ PAP, ↑ PAWP, ↓ CO, ↓ CI, ↓ O_2 saturation, ↑ SVR on hemodynamic monitoring

15. Diagnoses applicable at this time: Pain, Risk for impaired gas exchange, Ineffective management of therapeutic regime, Activity intolerance, Impaired skin integrity, Risk for altered role performance, PC: Pulmonary edema

Lesson 22 – Congestive Heart Failure—Part II: Thursday

1. Tuesday afternoon: Very worried about her condition; having difficulty breathing—possible CHF; patient and husband distraught about failing heart. Getting a CXR.
   Tuesday evening: Very tired; worried about how she will care for herself.
   Wednesday: Decreased pain; notation of generalized knowledge deficit regarding condition.

2. Physicians' orders:
   PA and lateral of chest stat
   Furosemide 20 mg IV stat; 40 mg PO qAM
   Chem 7 at 1900

3. CXR shows CHF with pleural effusions.

4. Cardiology report shows fluid overload; right-sided heart failure.

5. Table 22-1 Congestive Heart Failure

Subjective Data

Important Health Information

Past health history: CAD (including recent MI), hypertension, cardiomyopathy, valvular or congenital heart disease, diabetes mellitus, thyroid or lung disease, rapid or irregular heartbeat

Medications: Use of and compliance with any cardiac medications; use of diuretics, estrogens, corticosteroids, phenylbutazone, nonsteroidal antiinflammatory drugs

Functional Health Patterns

Health perception-health management: Fatigue

Nutritional-metabolic: Usual sodium intake; *nausea, vomiting, anorexia, *stomach bloating; weight gain

Elimination: Nocturia, decreased daytime urinary output, constipation

Activity-exercise: Dyspnea, orthopnea, cough; palpitations; dizziness, fainting

Sleep-rest: Number of pillows used for sleeping; paroxysmal nocturnal dyspnea

Cognitive-perceptual: Chest pain or heaviness; RUQ pain, *abdominal discomfort; behavioral changes

Objective Data

Integumentary

Cool, diaphoretic skin; cyanosis or pallor, *peripheral edema (right-sided heart failure)

Respiratory

*Tachypnea, *crackles, rhonchi, wheezes; frothy, blood-tinged sputum

Cardiovascular

*Tachycardia, *S_3, S_4, murmurs; pulsus alternans, PMI displaced inferiorly and posteriorly, *jugular vein distention

Gastrointestinal

*Abdominal distention, hepatosplenomegaly, ascites

Neurologic

*Restlessness, confusion, decreased attention or memory

Possible Findings

Altered serum electrolytes (especially Na^+ and K^+), elevated BUN, creatinine, or liver function tests; chest x-ray demonstrating cardiomegaly, pulmonary congestion, and interstitial pulmonary edema; echocardiogram showing increased chamber size and decreased wall motion; atrial and ventricular enlargement on ECG, $\uparrow$ PAP, $\uparrow$ PAWP, $\downarrow$ CO, $\downarrow$ CI, $\downarrow$ O_2 saturation, $\uparrow$ SVR on hemodynamic monitoring

6.

	Total Intake	Total Output
Sunday	570	250
Monday	3070	895
Tuesday through 1500	880	0
3-day totals	4520	1145

7. Carmen Gonzales was retaining fluid. Having no urine output at all on Tuesday through 1500 is a concern.

8. Fluid overload increases preload of the right side of the heart. Eventually the right side of the heart is unable to keep up with workload demands, and fluid literally backs up in the peripheral venous system, causing the symptoms described.

9. Furosemide works to reabsorb the sodium and chloride from the loop of Henle and distal renal tubule, which causes an increase of renal excretion of water.

10. Effect is diuresis and removal of excess fluid—relief of edema. This is measured by increased urine output and reduction of peripheral edema.

11. Very quick onset of action and very potent diuretic effects make furosemide the best choice in acute situations in which rapid diuresis is desired. IV route has faster onset and peak action than oral route. Thiazides are not available as IV meds; they are used for routine long-term diuresis.

12.

	Total Intake	Total Output
Sunday	570	250
Monday	3070	895
Tuesday	1595	1475
Wednesday	1215	1650
3-day totals	6450	4270

13. After the Lasix was given, the output increased significantly, thus reducing the fluid volume.

14.

Medication	Why Given	Time Due
Cefoxitin 2 g IVPB	Antibiotic to treat infection	0900 and 1500
Glyburide 3 mg PO qAM	Oral hypoglycemic to manage glucose levels	0800
Furosemide 40 mg PO qAM	Diuretic to reduce vascular volume	0800

15. Debridement 2 days ago; developed left-sided CHF from fluid volume overload. Was on diuretics to treat this. Lungs congested this morning. Slept well last night. No pain, no pain meds given. BP 145/80; RR 18–20; HR 75; oxygen sat 90%–95%. Blood glucose was 150 this morning.

16. Carmen Gonzales had right-sided CHF, not left-sided CHF.

17. Temperature: 98.6° F   Respiration: 20

   Heart rate: 84   Blood pressure: 146/98

   Pain rating: 1   Oxygen saturation: 94%

18. Previously Carmen Gonzales did not follow up with physician appointments after discharge.
   She does not seem knowledgeable about her disease process.
   Her lack of understanding about medication and diet therapy.
   Exercise at this point will be limited; will need to explore realistic options for this.
   Finances are limited.

19. Since her primary language is Spanish, a translator and patient teaching materials in Spanish must be provided.
   Must be sure to discuss dietary measures that are realistic for her to follow within her cultural norms.
   Must explore what her beliefs are regarding medication therapy.
   Explore her feelings and belief about medical care in general.

20. Note to the instructor: This sheet should be consistent with the information in Tables 33-10 and 33-11.

    What is a low-sodium diet?
    A low-sodium diet involves limiting salt in your diet. This means avoiding foods that contain a lot of salt. It is also important to not add salt to foods when preparing meals or while eating.

    Why is a low-sodium diet important for you to follow?
    Limiting the amount of salt in your food will help control excess fluid from accumulating in your body. This will in turn help to decrease how hard your heart has to work and will help to prevent the development of heart failure.

    Many of the foods that you currently enjoy can be included on this diet. They are:
    Chicken, pork, beans, etc.

    There are several foods that should be avoided, if possible, on this diet. Examples include:
    There are several items you can include here. Refer to Table 33-11 in your textbook.

21. Answers will vary tremendously. Probably the most important thing to include is the fact that Carmen Gonzales can continue to eat many of the same foods she has been eating. However she may have to modify how these foods are prepared.

Lesson 23 – Nutritional Problems

1. Candidiasis (patient can hardly swallow; has difficulty taking in food or fluid). Frequent throat and mouth infections. Ongoing poor appetite. Problems with diarrhea.

2. Metabolic needs associated with a chronic infection such as HIV significantly increase the metabolic rate. At the same time, problems such as anorexia, nausea, vomiting, and diarrhea make it difficult for patient to take in adequate calories.

3. Height: 6 feet 1 inch
   Weight 143 pounds

4. Body mass index is a height-to-weight ratio used to evaluate nutritional status. The normal range is 20–25.

5. BMI = 17

6. Ira Bradley is seriously underweight.

7. Albumin level.

8. Ira Bradley's albumin level: 2.1 g/dl
   Normal range: 3.5–5.0 g/dl

9. This indicates severe protein depletion.

10. Serum albumin level is useful in the diagnosis of malnutrition. The level for albumin reflects protein changes over the past several weeks, so it is not useful for acute changes in nutrition (changes in the last few days). Prealbumin level provides an indication of recent changes in nutritional status (i.e., over the past few days).

11. Each degree of temperature increase on the Fahrenheit scale raises BMR by 7%. Fever also increases insensible loss, thus increasing the fluid requirements.

12. Sunday 2400: 101.1° F   Monday 1200: 101.3° F

    Monday 0400: 101.1° F   Monday 1600: 101.4° F

    Monday 0800: 101.1° F   Monday 2000: 101.2° F

13. He has experienced a 14%–20% increase in BMR because his temperature has been about 2–3° F above normal range.

14. a. D_5 ½ NaCl @ 125 cc/hour

    b. D_5W has about 200 kcal/liter. ½ NaCl does not contain any kcals.

    c. About 3 liters

    d. Total calories from IV: 600 calories

    e. Ira Bradley's only intake was 25% of one meal on Monday evening. Estimated calories from meals (not including Tuesday's breakfast): 200 calories.

    f. Estimated total caloric intake (Sunday 2400 to Tuesday 0800): 800 calories

    g. Estimated caloric needs per 24 hours: 4500 calories.

    h. Net difference: –3700 calories

15. Ira Bradley has had very inadequate intake.

16. Over the course of the week, Ira Bradley begins to progressively increase his intake. By the end of the week, he is eating 100% of meals.

17. No. The nurse did not address this well at all. The only notation made in the nurses' notes regarding appetite or eating intake is on Wednesday.

18. These are collaborative measures, so obviously this would require a physicians' order. It is difficult to say whether more aggressive feeding should have been implemented because Ira Bradley is at "end stage" and there may be preestablished wishes regarding aggressive intervention. The risks and benefits must be weighed with all procedures. Given his end-stage condition, the patient may not want such aggressive measure done. It may also be possible that the risk for infection makes TPN too great a risk.

19. Answers will vary greatly, but should include frequent, small, high-calorie and high-protein meals, keeping in mind the foods Ira Bradley likes and those that he can easily eat.

Lesson 24 – Diabetes Mellitus—Part I: Tuesday

1. Decreased tissue responsiveness to insulin; overproduction of insulin early in the disease process with eventual decreased insulin secretion from beta cell exhaustion; and abnormal hepatic regulation.

2.

Character	Type 1 DM	Type 2 DM
Age of onset	Any age—usually during adolescence or young adulthood	Adult onset (usually over age 35)
Causes	Autoimmune disorder causing beta cell destruction	Obesity; familial tendencies
Symptoms at onset	Thirst, polyuria, fatigue, polyphagia	None or mild
Use of insulin	Must use insulin	May or may not need insulin—is used as supplement
Use of oral hypoglycemic agents	Not effective	Effective
Common complications	Multiple—all around vascular changes resulting in HTN, CAD, CHF, CRF, neuropathy, PVD, retinal changes, and more	Complications often less serious; however same problems can occur over time, especially with poor management

3. Chart mentions type 2 DM, CAD, family history of DM; last admission was related to DM; education was provided at that time.

4. Answers will vary significantly but should mention obtaining a blood sugar reading.

5. Coronary artery disease: Vascular complications—significant increased incidence of CAD.

Hypertension: Vascular complications—significant increase in HTN due to arteriosclerosis and atherosclerosis.

Congestive heart failure. Long-standing and poorly managed hypertension will eventually contribute to heart failure.

Infection to leg: Diseased blood vessels result in poor microcirculation—leads to peripheral vascular disease and risk for ulcers and infection.

6.

Clinical Picture	Textbook Description	Carmen Gonzales' Data	Fits Description? (Yes or No)
Age of onset	Age 35 or older, but half of cases occur in people over 55.	Unknown age of diagnosis; she is 56 years old.	Yes
Ethnicity	Highest incidence in Native Americans; occurrence in Hispanic population two times higher than in non-Hispanic whites.	Hispanic	Yes
Obesity	Normal weight to obese	5 feet 2 inches; weighs 170 pounds BMI = 31 (obese)	Yes
Familial factors	Familial tendencies, but no specific genetic link	Possibility that mother had DM	Yes

7. Glyburide 3 mg PO qd
   ADA 1500-calorie diet
   Monitor blood glucose levels AC and HS
   Sliding scale insulin order

8. 4 doses of insulin (6 units, 4 units, and 2 units twice).

9. Since Carmen Gonzales has type 2 DM, she produces insulin and the oral hypoglycemic agent helps to stimulate the release of the insulin. With the stress of illness, glucose levels tend to increase; also, infection and stress typically alter the requirements for control of blood sugar, and she may be unable to produce adequate amounts of insulin to meet her needs. For this reason, supplemental insulin is given based on her glucose levels.

10. Generic name: Glyburide

    Common trade names: DiaBeta, Micronase

    Mechanisms of action: Stimulates the release of insulin from the pancreas and increases sensitivity to insulin at receptor sites

    Dosage: Varies with each individual; ranges from 1.25–20 mg/day

    Administration routes: Only administered orally

11.

Medication	**Why Given**	**Time Due**
Cefoxitin 2 g IVPB	Antibiotic to treat infection	0900 1500
Glyburide 3 mg PO qAM	Oral hypoglycemic agent used to manage glucose levels	0800

12. At midnight her glucose level was 190. She was administered 2 units of regular insulin.

13. Carmen Gonzales had a pain rating of 8; therefore it would be appropriate to give her a pain medication at this time.

14. Sulfonylureas are ideally administered with meals for optimal diabetic control and to minimize gastric irritation. Compliance will be higher if patients do not experience the side effect of gastric irritation.

15.

	Expected Length of Time	**Actual Time After 0730 Dose**
Onset	30–60 minutes	0800–0830
Peak	2–4 hours	0930–1130
Duration	6 hours	1330

16. **Head and Neck**
    PERRLA; 3-mm pupils; oral mucosa dry
    Nares without drainage; mucosa dry
    2+ carotid pulse; no JVD noted

Chest/Upper Extremities

Chest expansion equal; bilateral crackles auscultated; productive cough
S_1 and S_2 noted; no murmurs
Radial pulses 2+; no edema in upper extremities
Cap refill <3 sec; hand strength bilaterally equal

Abdomen and Lower Extremities

Bowel sounds auscultated 4 quadrants
Abdomen soft, round, no tenderness
Dorsalis pedis +1L +2R
Edema 1+ bilaterally in legs
Wound on lower left leg

17. Answers will vary. Findings are consistent with previous findings by nurses, except possibly edema in legs.

Lesson 25 – Diabetes Mellitus—Part II: Thursday

1.

Medication	Why Given	Time Due
Cefoxitin 2 g IVPB	Antibiotic to treat infection	0900 and 1500
Glyburide 3 mg PO qAM	Oral hypoglycemic to manage glucose levels	0800
Furosemide 40 mg PO qAM	Diuretic to reduce vascular volume	0800

2. Lasix was given because Carmen Gonzales developed right-sided CHF on Tuesday afternoon. Lasix is being given to control excess fluid. Furosemide has the potential to cause elevations in glucose levels.

3. Nurse talked about her pain level, her vitals, and her CHF episode yesterday. Only mention of DM was this morning's blood glucose level. No mention of stability of glucose levels or need for insulin.

4. Heart rate: 82
   Respiration: 19
   Blood pressure: 145/80
   Temperature: 98.6
   Oxygen saturation: 94%
   Pain rating: 1

5. Perception/Self-Concept: Is afraid she can't walk; cannot do anything because leg hurts. Does not feel well; feel hopeless.

   Activity: Works at senior citizen center part-time preparing meals; at this time, can't do much. Watches TV and goes to bed; husband has to help a lot; sometimes youngest daughter helps as well.

   Sexuality/Reproductive: Says, "Too old for that." Still hugs a lot; has two grown children; daughter lives with them at home right now.

   Culture: Parents from Mexico; speaks Spanish and English; considers herself American.

   Nutrition-Metabolic: Still has her own teeth; no dentures/bridges; does admit to recent toothaches. Usually eats eggs, beans, potatoes. Likes chicken, rice, BBQ pork, tortillas. Eats few vegetables/fruits. No change in weight.

Sleep-Rest: Pain interferes with sleep; feels tired all the time.

Role/Relationship: Close family; has friends at senior citizen center; gets along well with them; no other friends mentioned. Unable to work right now.

Health Perception: Feels health is out of her control; getting sicker and sicker. Eats her own way; will try to control diabetes.

Elimination: No problems.

Cognitive/Perceptual: No difficulty with language or memory. Some changes in vision. Decisions about care on discharge: plans to have daughter move in and take care of her and husband.

Coping/Stress: Daughter will be at home to help. Other support systems: friends at senior citizen center will bring food.

Value/Belief: Values family. Priest came to visit; reads Bible. Friends and work very important.

6. Despite previous DM teaching, Carmen Gonzales does not seem knowledgeable about her disease process.

   Lack of understanding about medication and diet therapy.

   Exercise at this point will be limited; will need to explore realistic options for this.

   Finances are limited.

   Has daughter may help care for her.

7. Since her primary language is Spanish, a translator and patient teaching materials in Spanish must be provided.

   Must be sure to discuss dietary measures that are realistic for her to follow within her cultural norms.

   Must explore what her beliefs are regarding medication therapy.

8. Answers will vary.

9. One of the most challenging obstacles is getting the patient to understand and value the importance of nutrition control, as well as seeing that she has assistance in her daily activities.

10. Answers will vary.

Lesson 26 – Closed Head Injury

1. David Ruskin was thrown headfirst off his bicycle after being hit by an automobile. He struck a post; he was wearing a helmet; the helmet was cracked from the impact. He had LOC. He then woke up and was walking around at the accident scene.

2. David Ruskin was oriented to person, but not to place or time. Glascow = 12; PERRLA with 3-mm pupils.

3. The Glascow Coma Scale is a method to assess level of consciousness with a universal scoring system. The score applies to three areas: eye opening, verbal response, and motor response. David Ruskin's score is 12. This means he has deficits worth 3 points; however the score does not tell us where his deficits are. Coma is 8 or below.

4. Head injury can trigger three possible events leading to cerebral edema: hemorrhage, contusion, and posttraumatic brain swelling.

5. a. Cerebral edema results in increased tissue volume. The increased volume within the closed skull cavity leads to increase in pressure.

   b. Increased ICP leads to a decrease in cerebral perfusion due to compression of the blood vessels. If there is a decrease in perfusion, there is a decrease in oxygenation to the brain tissue, and ischemia occurs, further causing edema. Decreased oxygen leads to an accumulation of CO_2, which causes a vasodilation of the blood vessels; this then leads to further increased ICP because of increased blood volume flowing through the vessels.

6. High-flow oxygen helps to reduce the build-up of CO_2. Since CO_2 levels cause vasodilation, build-up makes the potential for increased ICP greater.

7. Headache, change or decrease in level of consciousness, nausea, vomiting.

8. CT scan: Performed to detect problems such as hemorrhage or edema.

   Skull series: Performed to detect fractures. This would be evident on CT scan as well.

9. Both tests were negative.

10. The patient must lie very still—this is difficult for disoriented patients. A very short-acting sedative can be given to facilitate this procedure.

11. Admit ICU for observation CHI.
    Monitor vital signs and neuro checks q 1 hour × 4 hours; then q 2 hours.

12. Vital signs may give indication of changes in ICP. With increased ICP, the blood pressure increases with a slowing of the heart rate. Changes in respiratory patterns may also indicate changes in ICP.

13. Neurologic checks would include the following:
    Glascow Coma Scale
    Pupil size and response
    Mental status assessment (person, place, time, behavior)
    Other cranial nerve checks as appropriate
    Could also include motor system exam to assess gait, symmetric movement, strength, and fine motor skills.
    (Note: CMS check should not be listed here—this is to assess circulation and movement of the arm.)

14. Status has changed a little—from GCS of 15 and full level of orientation immediately post-op to GCS of 14 with some disorientation on Monday afternoon. Nurse indicates possibility of medications causing slight disorientation.

15. The only report information related to the CHI is that he hit his head and was in ICU. No update on neuro status is given.

16. The nurses are supposed to be performing neuro checks. Some information related to this should have been included.

17. Temperature: 99.1° F

    Blood pressure: 126/68

    Heart rate: 78

    Respiration: 20

    Oxygen saturation: 91%

    Pain rating: 5

18. Mental status: Is awake and alert—time orientation seems OK based on history

    Pupil response/size: Pupils checked—PERRLA, 3-mm pupils

    Glascow Coma Scale: 15

    Motor strength: Weakness to right hand (fracture)

    Other cranial nerves assessed: Six cardinal fields of gaze assessed—evaluates CN III, IV, and VI

19. Epidural hematoma: Unlikely

    Acute subdural hematoma: Unlikely

    Subacute subdural hematoma: Likely

20. Subacute subdural hematoma can occur 48 hours to 2 weeks after the initial injury. Symptoms will include general deterioration of mental status several days after a closed head injury. This type of problem may not be detectable by the CT scan immediately after the injury.

Lesson 27 – Acute Spinal Cord Injury—Part 1: Preclinical Preparation

1. Diving board accident. She flipped off a board and landed against the concrete edge of swimming pool.

2. Pupils: PERRLA, pupils 3-mm

    Glasgow Coma Scale: 15

    Orientation: OR × 4

    Cranial nerves: CN 2–12 all intact

    Peripheral nerves: Movement/sensation in upper extremities; no sensation below nipple line; unable to move lower extremities; deep tendon reflexes in lower extremities hyperactive; flaccid paralysis below nipple line

3. Burst fracture of T6, fractured posterior 6th rib. The MRI shows a partially transected spinal cord.

4. Injury in the cord cause hemorrhages in the central gray matter of the cord. The hemorrhage and edema cause ischemia to the cord tissue; this progresses to necrosis of the tissue because of lack of oxygen in the tissue. Necrosis of the cord results essentially in a loss of the affected tissue and loss of function below the level of the lesion.

5. Spinal edema contributes to the cord ischemia.

6.

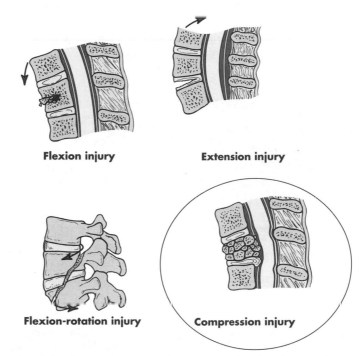

Flexion injury   **Extension injury**

Flexion-rotation injury   **Compression injury**

7. A partial transection (also known as *incomplete cord lesion involvement*) occurs when the cord is damaged but not completely severed. With this type of lesion, there is a mixed loss of voluntary motor activity and sensation—some tracts are left intact.

8. Central cord syndrome, anterior cord syndrome, Brown-Sequard syndrome, and posterior cord syndrome

9. It is unlikely she has central cord syndrome—this is usually associated with injury in older adults who have osteoarthritis in the spine.

   Brown-Sequard is also unlikely—this is usually associated with a penetrating injury such as a knife or gunshot wound.

   Anterior cord syndrome or posterior cord syndrome are both possible. Anterior cord syndrome is associated with acute hyperflexion injury; posterior cord syndrome is associated with acute hyperextension injury. Although anterior cord syndrome is more common, both are possibilities with a diving accident.

10. Spinal shock is characterized by decreased reflexes and flaccid paralysis below the level of the injury. This usually occurs at the time of injury in response to the severe damage to the cord. It usually lasts for 7 to 10 days after the onset, but it can last for weeks to months. After spinal shock has resolved, one can determine the degree of actual paralysis from the injury.

11. While the patient is in spinal shock, the bladder is atonic and becomes overdistended. An indwelling catheter is inserted to drain the bladder.

12.

Drug	Typical Dose and Administration	Beneficial Effects
Administration of methyl-prednisolone is considered standard care for acute spinal cord injury.	30 mg/kg bolus in 15 minutes. Follow 45 minutes later with continuous infusion 5.4 mg/kg/hour for 23 hours.	MP has been found to improve blood flow and reduce edema in the spinal spinal cord, thus reducing cord ischemia.

13. It was necessary to alleviate compression of the spine, which was potentially limiting circulation to the cord. Also, there was a need to stabilize the spine to prevent further injury.

14.

Orders (not including medications)	Rationale
Oxygen per nasal cannula; keep O_2 sat >90%	She has a risk for impaired gas exchange because of her immobility as well as potential respiratory muscle involvement. Oxygen helps to maintain oxygenation to peripheral tissues.
Pulmonary toilet q4h	She has a risk for impaired gas exchange because of her immobility as well as potential respiratory muscle involvement. She will need aggressive deep breathing and coughing exercises to minimize her risk.
Compression gradient stockings; remove for 30 minutes q8h	She has a risk for deep vein thrombosis because of venous pooling associated with the spinal cord injury. The stockings should be removed every shift to assess skin.
Heel protectors	She has a huge risk for skin breakdown; heels are particularly a problem because this is a natural pressure point while in bed.
I&O q8h	It is important to monitor the intake and output to evaluate adequacy of fluid intake. Additionally, bladder distention may occur; output measurement may help recognize this.
Diet/tolerated; encourage high-protein, high-carbohydrate, high-calorie, high-fiber diet.	There in an increased metabolic demand after this type of injury; additionally, appetite is frequently reduced. High carbohydrates and proteins are ideal for rehabilitation. High-fiber diet will help to minimize the problems associated with constipation.

15. | **Medication** | **Classification** | **Reason Given** |
|---|---|---|
| Famotidine 20 mg PO q12h | H$_2$ inhibitor | Given as prophylactic agent to prevent stress ulcer. |
| Docusate Sodium 100 mg PO QD | Laxative | She is at risk for constipation—given to prevent this. |
| Biscodyl suppository PRN QD | Laxative | She is at risk for constipation—given to prevent this. |
| Multiple vitamin with minerals qAM | Vitamin supplement | Given to help maintain adequate nutrition; common for poor appetite following SCI. Will help with healing. |
| Vitamin C 500 mg PO qPM | Vitamin supplement | Given to help maintain adequate nutrition; common for poor appetite following SCI. Will help with healing process |
| Enoxaparin 30 mg SC q12h | Anticoagulant (low-molecular–weight heparin) | Prevention of deep vein thrombosis and pulmonary emboli—she is at risk for these because of immobility and venous pooling. |
| Baclofen 10 mg PO q12h | Skeletal muscle relaxant | Indicated for treatment of spasticity associated with spinal cord injury. |
| Acetaminophen 600 mg PO PRN | Antipyretic, analgesic | Ordered for mild pain or for fever. |
| Oxycodone/acetaminophen 1 tablet PO PRN | Opioid analgesic | Ordered for more severe pain the patient may be experiencing. |

16. a. Concerns:
     Patient's concern regarding loss of body function and perceived expectations
     Skin breakdown
     Autonomic dysreflexia
     Pneumonia
     DVT/PE
     Family adjustment
     Grieving

   b. Problem list (nursing diagnoses and collaborative problems):
     Body image disturbance
     Risk for impaired tissue integrity
     Impaired mobility
     Risk for ineffective coping (individual and family)
     PC: DVT
     PC: PE
     PC: Stasis pneumonia
     PC: Autonomic dysreflexia

Lesson 28 – Acute Spinal Cord Injury—Part II

1. Transection of T5; arrived on floor on Monday after 1 week in ICU; vitals are stable; awake and oriented; oxygen sat 90–92 on room air; lungs clear; heart sounds normal; peripheral circulation OK.

   Indication that family members are present but have not spent a lot of time in the room.

2. Original report said T6 partial transection. No mention was made about incision site; this may have been appropriate.

3. Heart rate: 60   Temperature: 99° F

   Respiratory rate: 20   Oxygen Saturation: 92%

   Blood pressure: 90/62   Pain Scale/Location: 9

4. Andrea Wang has pain of 9/10 and is complaining of headache. She should be medicated with hydrocodone/acetaminophen.

5. **Head and Neck**
   Oculomoter function intact; PERRLA; 21-mm pupils.
   Oral mucosa moist, nares clear. No lymphadenopathy. Range of motion in neck without pain. Carotid pulse +2.

   Chest/Upper Extremities
   Chest symmetrical with equal expansion.
   S_1 and S_2 heart sounds normal.
   Lungs clear but diminished in the bases; chest excursion within defined limits; crackles in bases.
   Radial pulses +2; cap refill <3 sec.

   Abdomen and Lower Extremities
   Bowel sounds × 4.
   Foley catheter present; clear yellow urine.
   Pulses in dorsalis pedis 2+ left; 3+ right.
   Pulses in posterior tibialis 1+ left; 2+ right.

6. Order calls for enoxaparin 30 mg, SQ.

7. Perception/Self-Concept: Feeling overwhelmed; wants to go back to school; worried about boyfriend's perception; not dealing well with problem.

   Activity: Full-time student; works part-time jobs; recreation—water sports; helps to take care of parents; wants to go back to school and be able to help parents.

   Sexuality/Reproduction: Sexually active with boyfriend (live together); is worried about impact of injury on this relationship.

   Culture: Chinese American—identity is Asian American; only language is English.

   Nutrition-Metabolic: Eats OK; teeth OK; no problems.

   Sleep-Rest: Not sleeping well at hospital; sleeping off and on; feels exhausted and helpless.

   Role/Relationship: Family is close; has brother and sister who live in another city for school; has lots of friends; goes out a lot; works as waitress and at ski resort.

Health Perception: Good health; never sick; does not know what plan is; can't imagine self in a wheelchair; learns best by talking and demonstration.

Elimination: Incontinent now; very worried about this.

Cognitive/Perceptual: Understands everything; has good memory; no change in vision or hearing.

Coping/Stress: Family not working things out; does not depend on parents; boyfriend is only support aside from parents; parents need help with care. Feeling overwhelmed.

Value/Belief: Not very religious; could not connect with priest; does not practice religion. Family/parents/boyfriend do not know what will happen in future.

8. Obviously, this list will vary from student to student, but here is the author's suggested list:

Original Problem List (from Lesson 27)	**New Revised Problem List**
Nursing diagnoses:	Nursing diagnoses:
Body image disturbance	Body image disturbance
Risk for impaired tissue integrity	Risk for impaired tissue integrity
Impaired mobility	Impaired mobility
Risk for constipation	Risk for constipation
Risk for ineffective airway clearance	Ineffective coping (individual and family)
	Sexual dysfunction
	Pain
	Sleep pattern disturbance
	Risk for ineffective role performance
Collaborative problems:	Collaborative problems:
PC: DVT	PC: DVT
PC: PE	PC: PE
PC: Stasis pneumonia	PC: Stasis pneumonia
PC: Autonomic dysreflexia	PC: Autonomic dysreflexia

9. Was very restless during the night; had nausea, headache, blurred vision; was coherent and oriented × 3; vitals stable; oxygen saturation >92% all night.

10. **Case Manager**
Four major concerns:
   Ineffective coping, individual and family
   Integration of nursing and rehabilitative care
   Inadequate social support
   Monitoring for complications associated with SCI

Social Worker
Two major concerns:
   Family coping
   Sexuality

Clinical Nurse Specialist
Spinal shock seems to be resolving. Focus on possibility of autonomic dysreflexia, respiratory compromise, DVT, infection, and skin breakdown.

11. Autonomic dysreflexia is an uncompensated cardiovascular reaction mediated by the SNS. It occurs in response to visceral stimulation once spinal shock is resolved in patients with spinal cord injuries above T7. The most common cause is a distended bladder; stimulation of pain receptors, skin, or contraction of the rectum can also stimulate this.

    The pathology involves stimulation of the sensory receptors below the level of SCI. This stimulation causes vasoconstriction, leading to hypertension. This stimulates parasympathetic system, causing bradycardia. Symptoms include sudden acute headache, flushed face, sweating above level of injury, apprehension.

    This is an emergency situation. Immediate interventions are to elevate head of bed 45 degrees, relieve the source of the stimulation, and contact primary care provider immediately.

12. Poor appetite and decreased food intake
    Restlessness/headache during night
    Getting ready for transfer to rehabilitation

13. Change position frequently: if in a w/c, lift self up and shift weight every 15 to 30 minutes; if in bed, get on a regular turning schedule—change position minimum of every 2 hours.
    Use pillows to protect bony prominences.
    Use special mattresses and wheelchair cushions.
    Inspect skin frequently for evidence of skin breakdown.

14. Autonomic dysreflexia

15. Kinked catheter

16. Yes—headache, blurred vision, nauseated, hypertensive, flushed face.

Lesson 29 – Skeletal Fracture

1. Edema: Excessive edema can impair circulation if not controlled.

    Decreased function: Lack of function is one of the more common indicators of fracture.

    (Pain:) Pain encourages splinting of fractured extremity.

    Ecchymosis: Bruising usually does not become evident for several days following an injury.

    Crepitation: This finding typically indicates a nonunion of the bone and an unstable fracture.

2. The ER report includes very little data regarding the fracture—only additional finding is the x-ray report indicating comminuted fracture.

3. Distal pulses
   Paresthesia
   Color (pallor)
   Pain
   Paralysis

    You would also want to assess and document overall appearance (deformity) and warmth.

4.

Presenting Injury	Priority of Assessment	Impact of Injury on Assessment of the Arm (if any)
Closed head injury	1	May make it more difficult to get reliable history and assessment with change in mental status
Laceration	3	None
Fractured right arm	2	N/A
Abrasions to right flank and calf	4	May give clues as to impact on right side of body

5. Comminuted

6.

Medication	Why Given	Time Due
Cefoxitin 1 g IVPB q6h	Prevention of infection	0900
Oxycodone 5–10 mg PO q4h PRN moderate pain	Pain management	PRN—no schedule
Acetaminophen	Mild pain management or temperature	PRN—no schedule

7. Had ORIF on Sunday; stable vitals, slight temp; oriented to person/place; IV L hand without swelling; slight pain with breathing; abrasions to left side.

8. Nurse reported left arm pain and left-side abrasions; chart clearly indicates these occur on right. Nurse did not indicate CMS checks.

9. Risk for peripheral nerve dysfunction: CMS checks, elevation; monitor for development (escalating pain, edema, loss of function, and sensation).

Pain: Elevation, ice, pain medications.

Risk for infection: Handwashing, aseptic technique, antibiotic administration. Monitor for development of infection (fever, incision, etc).

PC: Fat embolus: Monitor for development of complication.

10. Heart rate: 78   Temperature: 99.1° F

Respiratory rate: 20   Oxygen saturation: 91%

Blood pressure: 126/68

11. **Head and Neck**

PEERLA; 3-mm pupils; 6 cardinal fields of gaze.

Oral mucosa pink, dry without lesions; nares dry, clear passages, no drainage; no lymphadenopathy.

Oriented to person and place; confused to time.

Chest/Upper Extremities

Respirations unlabored; chest wall equal expansion; bilaterally symmetrical. Lungs clear in all lung fields; S_1 and S_2 heart sounds auscultated.

Radial pulses equal bilaterally 2+; cap refill <3 sec.

Abdomen and Lower Extremities

Bowel sounds faint; abdomen flat, firm; no tenderness or masses.

Dorsalis pedis and posterior tibialis pulses equal bilaterally. Cap refill <3 sec. No edema.

12. David Ruskin needs to have his arm elevated on a sky hook or on a pillow.

13. Pain rating = 7/10

    Medication(s) available: Oxycodone 5 to 10 mg or acetaminophen

    Other symptoms: Pain is sharp in chest—worse with breathing.

    Decision: Medicate David Ruskin with 5 mg oxycodone.

    Rationale: Since his pain is 7/10 (moderate pain), oxycodone is best choice. Has not had any pain medication since 0400; was given 5 mg last dose.

14. Prevention of infection from surgery

15. Dextrose and saline solutions

16. 15 to 30 minutes

17. 13,000

18. It could mean infection. The WBC could also be elevated from the stress of the injury and surgery.

19. He has been running a steady low-grade fever.

20. These can be checked to monitor for therapeutic effect of the drug.

Lesson 30 – Osteomyelitis

1. Infection of the bone

2. *Acute osteomyelitis* refers to initial infection or an infection less than 1 month in duration.

   Chronic osteomyelitis refers to a bone infection that persists longer than 1 month or an infection that fails to respond to initial course of treatment.

3. Direct invasion: Contamination as a result of an open fracture or surgery.

   Indirect invasion: Contamination results from a blood-borne infection from a distant site such as teeth, infected tonsils, diabetic ulcers, or furuncles.

4. **Local Symptoms**   **Systemic Symptoms**

Local Symptoms	Systemic Symptoms
Swelling	Fever
Warmth at infection site	Nausea
Restricted movement	Malaise

5. Type of invasion: Indirect
   Identify Source: Diabetic ulcer—wound infection

6. Correct order of answers is as follows:

No	b	MRI and CT scan
Yes	a	Wound culture
No	d	Blood leukocyte count
Yes	f	X-ray of affected extremity
No	e	Radionuclide bone scan
No	c	Bone/tissue biopsy

7. Finding documented on the x-ray report: "Periosteal elevation on the left tissue."

   Meaning: The infection causes a pressure in the bone and causes ischemia to the bone.
   Ischemia causes area of the bone to die; sequestra forms in the area.
   The area of sequestra eventually enlarges and shows as an elevation area on x-ray. Keep in
   mind that if the x-ray reveals osteomyelitis, the disease is probably progressed.

8. Surgical debridement of the wound was done, but it was limited to gangrenous necrotic soft
   tissue. There is no indication of bony debridement.

9.

Medication	Why Given	Time Due
Cefoxitin 2 g IVPB	Antibiotic to treat infection	0900 and 1500
Glyburide 3 mg PO qAM	Oral hypoglycemic to manage glucose levels	0800
D_5W 100 cc/hour	Hydration	Continuous

10.

Test	Result	What does this mean?
Hgb	11.4 g/dl	This is a little low. She may be anemic.
Hct	33.6%	This is a little low. She may be anemic.
WBC	18.2	Normal is about 10. This is elevated—indicates an infection.

11. Type 2 DM; gangrene to left leg; surgical debridement yesterday. Elevated BP last night; hx
    of CHF, "keep eye on her"; oxygen sats OK; received pain medication 5 mg MS IM at 2300
    last night—no other pain.

12. Report could have been a bit more informative. Did not indicate how much insulin given
    and at what time; did not indicate what, if anything, has been done about the hypertension
    during the night. Very little mention was made about osteomyelitis—could have commented
    on the dressing/wound data.

13. Heart rate—92
    Respiratory rate—24
    Blood pressure—148/92

    Temperature—99° F
    Oxygen saturation—91%
    Pain rating—8

14. Carmen Gonzales had a pain rating of 8; therefore a pain medication is appropriate.

15. Yes. It is compatible with dextrose and saline solutions.

16. Run in over 15 to 30 minutes.

17. 100–200 cc/hour

18. Answers will vary.

19. Wound care instructions, IV antibiotic therapy, follow-up lab testing